BRITISH MEDICAL ASSOCIATION
Board of Science and Education

EATING DISORDERS, BODY IMAGE & THE MEDIA

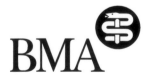

May 2000

Editorial Board

A publication from the BMA Board of Science and Education and the BMA Science Department:

Chairman, Board of Science and Education: Sir William Asscher

Head of Professional Resources and
   Research Group: Professor Vivienne Nathanson

Editor: Dr David R Morgan

Researched and Written by: Marcia Darvell

Contributing Authors (Steering Group): Dr Ahmed Elsharkawy[1]
Dr Jason C G Halford[2]
Dr Andrew J Hill[3]
Dr Jane Richards[4]
Dr Philip Steadman[5]

Editorial Secretariat: Laura Conway
Dawn Whyndham

Design: Hilary Forrester

First published in 2000 by: British Medical Association
BMA House
Tavistock Square
London WC1H 9JP

British Library Cataloguing-in-Publication Data
A catalogue record for this book is available from the British Library

ISBN: 0 7279 15339

Cover Photo: Telegraph Colour Library

Printed by: The Chameleon Press Limited

[1] Member, BMA Board of Science and Education
[2] Lecturer in Human Ingestive Behaviour, Department of Psychology, University of Liverpool
[3] Senior Lecturer in Behavioural Sciences, Academic Unit of Psychiatry and Behavioural Sciences, University of Leeds
[4] Member, BMA Board of Science and Education
[5] Deputy Member, BMA Board of Science and Education

Board of Science and Education

This report was prepared under the auspices of the Board of Science and Education of the British Medical Association, whose membership for 1999/00 was as follows:

Sir Peter Froggatt — President, BMA
Professor B R Hopkinson — Chairman, Representative Body
Dr I G Bogle — Chairman, BMA Council
Dr W J Appleyard — Treasurer, BMA
Sir William Asscher — Chairman, Board of Science and Education
Dr P H Dangerfield — Deputy Chairman, Board of Science and Education

Dr A Elsharkawy
Dr H W K Fell
Dr R Gupta (Deputy)
Dr S Hajioff
Dr V Leach
Dr N D L Olsen
Professor M R Rees
Dr S J Richards
Miss S Somjee
Dr P Steadman (Deputy)
Dr S Taylor
Dr D M B Ward

Approval for publication as a BMA policy report was recommended by BMA Executive Committee of Council on 19 April 2000.

Acknowledgements

The Association is pleased to acknowledge the help provided by many individuals and organisations in the preparation of this document and is extremely grateful for the guidance provided by the BMA Craft Committees, and Members of Council. We would also like to thank Dr Cindy Carter, Mr Roger Dickinson, and Professor Gerald Russell for their expert help.

Contents

Foreword by Dr Ian Bogle

Eating disorders have one of the highest mortality rates of all psychiatric illnesses, and are an increasing problem in modern Western societies. Anorexia nervosa and bulimia nervosa predominantly affect young women, and can have serious medical consequences that are often fatal. The disease does not just affect the individual sufferer, but can have a profound impact upon all family members. Parents, for example, may experience guilt, desperation, anger or fear, and will often blame themselves for the development of eating disorders in their children.

From a clinical perspective, it is important that individual sufferers of anorexia and bulimia nervosa are encouraged to see their general practitioner as soon as possible, since early diagnosis and treatment can make a significant contribution to the likelihood of an early recovery. Eating disorders are secretive illnesses. Many patients deny being ill and resist offers of help. It is, therefore, important that parents and carers learn to recognise early symptoms of eating disorders in young people, and encourage them to seek medical help (a list of symptoms can be found in Annex One). Self-help groups such as the Eating Disorders Association can provide additional information, confidential advice and support to sufferers (see Annex Four).

There are many treatments for eating disorders — behavioural, cognitive and pharmacological, which can often lead to complete recovery. However, long-term mortality and morbidity from eating disorders remains high, and can have long-lasting effects on the health of young people. The primary prevention of eating disorders is a priority. If, as a society, we can identify risk factors that may trigger eating disorders in vulnerable individuals, then we may be able to reduce the number of young people who develop eating disorders.

This British Medical Association report is not intended to be a guide to the diagnosis and treatment of eating disorders, but considers the risk factor of the media. The report considers the role of the media in perpetuating body dissatisfaction, especially in young women, and triggering eating disorders in vulnerable individuals. The mass media provide major sources of enjoyment, education and conversation in contemporary society, but also present us with unobtainable images of bodily perfection which can adversely effect the self-esteem and dieting behaviour of young women. Research shows that female models are becoming thinner at a time when women are becoming heavier, and the gap between the 'ideal' body shape and the reality is wider than ever. There is a need for more realistic body shapes to be shown on television and in fashion magazines, and to reduce young women's exposure to extremely thin models. We should also provide children and young people with the skills and information to resist media messages of bodily perfection.

This report reviews the evidence of media effects on self-esteem, body image and eating disorders, and aims to raise awareness of this important public health issue, with recommendations for action by government, media and education professionals, healthcare staff and others. I hope that urgent action will be taken to reduce the pressure on young women to be thin, and to reduce the number of young people who develop anorexia and bulimia nervosa.

Dr Ian Bogle
Chairman of Council
BMA

Introduction

The British Medical Association (BMA) is the professional organisation representing doctors in the UK. It was established in 1832 to "promote the medical and allied sciences, and to maintain the honour and interests of the profession". The Board of Science and Education, a standing committee of the Association, supports this aim by acting as an interface between the profession, the government and public, and by undertaking research studies on behalf of the BMA. Through the publication of policy statements, the Board of Science and Education has led the debate on key public health and professional issues. The Board has published a large number of reports over recent years reflecting current concerns in public health, such as *Growing up in Britain: ensuring a healthy future for our children* (1999); *The Impact of Genetic Modification on Agriculture, Food and Health* (1999); *Alcohol and Young People* (1999); *Domestic Violence: a health care issue?* (1998); *Road Transport and Health* (1997); and *Therapeutic Uses of Cannabis* (1997). Many of these publications illustrate the important links between wider social policy initiatives and good health care outcomes, and reflect the view that "Health is a state of complete physical, mental and social well-being, not merely the absence of disease and infirmity"(WHO 1946). The BMA, therefore, not only consider issues relating to clinical care and efficacy, but also examines the wider influences in society on the individual's health and well-being.

At the British Medical Association's 1998 Annual Representative Meeting the following resolution was passed and referred to the Board of Science and Education: *"That this meeting fears that some forms of advertising may be contributing to an increase in the incidence and prevalence of anorexia nervosa. It calls for greater responsibility in the use of such images in the media".*

The resolution was considered by the Board of Science and Education in April 1999 and members decided to review the wider influence of the media on self-esteem and body image perceptions in contemporary Western industrialised culture, especially in relation to the onset of eating disorders in vulnerable individuals, both male and female. In preparing its report, the Board decided to concentrate on the eating disorders of anorexia nervosa and bulimia nervosa, and not to include an analysis of issues related to obesity.

This report considers the role the media can play in shaping young people's attitudes to eating and body shape, and developing self-esteem in the young

3

who are at the greatest risk of developing an eating disorder. The report will consider whether the media play a significant role in the causation of eating disorders, where they can 'trigger' the illness in vulnerable individuals by suggesting that being 'thin' means being successful, and how they affect young people who may have low self-esteem or unhealthy attitudes towards food. More positively, the media may be able to significantly contribute towards developing high self-esteem in young people, and actively participate in health promotion to combat the mistaken belief that "thin = healthy" and that 'dieting' rather than healthy eating and regular exercise, is the way to achieve a healthy weight.

This report concentrates on sociocultural trends which may contribute to the onset of eating disorders, and does not differentiate between anorexia nervosa and bulimia nervosa in considering eating disorders as a public health issue since about 40-50% of most severely bulimic patients have a history of anorexia nervosa.[1,2] Also, many of the arguments about the media's effect on self-esteem, body image and eating behaviour apply equally to both conditions[3] — both have serious health consequences. For ease of description the term 'eating disorders' will often be used to refer to both anorexia and bulimia nervosa.

Anorexia and bulimia nervosa: clinical descriptions

The American Psychiatric Association's Diagnostic and Statistical Manual of Mental Disorders (DSM IV)[4] provides definitions of anorexia nervosa and bulimia nervosa (see Annex Two). In this criteria, anorexia nervosa is characterised by deliberate weight loss, leading to a body weight that is at least 15% below the normal or expected weight for height or age (body weight is usually judged by the Body Mass Index, discussed on page 14). The weight loss is self-induced by avoiding foods which are perceived to be fattening. There is a self-perception of fatness and hormonal disturbance which can lead to amenorrhoea (lack of menstruation) in women and a loss of sexual potency in men.[5] The illness generally begins in early adolescence, between the ages of 13 and 18 years.[4]

Bulimia nervosa is diagnosed by the presence of binge eating, where there are recurrent episodes of over-eating at least twice a week over a period of three months, and inappropriate compensatory behaviours to prevent weight gain (eg self-induced vomiting, misuse of laxatives, diuretics, or other medications, fasting or excessive exercise). Bulimia nervosa tends to have a later age of onset than anorexia nervosa.[4] Both bulimia nervosa and anorexia nervosa can result in serious medical complications. It should be noted that anorexia nervosa can affect elderly people.[6] It has been suggested that the condition may be underdiagnosed in postmenopausal women[7] and should be considered in the diagnosis of an elderly patient presenting with unexplained weight loss.[6] However, the disorder rarely occurs in females over the age of 40.[4] This report will concentrate on young women (who comprise the majority of eating disorder sufferers,) and who are most likely to be exposed to the risk factor of particular forms of the media (eg fashion advertising).

Eating disorders are a significant cause of mortality and morbidity in young people in modern industrialised societies. Health complications suffered by individuals with anorexia and bulimia nervosa include the following areas of illness and disability:[8]

- Cardiovascular (eg abnormal heart rhythm, hypotension, cardiac failure);

- Skeletal (eg osteoporosis, pathological fractures);

- Gastrointestinal (eg erosion of dental enamel, peptic ulcers, delayed gastric emptying);

- Renal (increased blood urea, electrolytic abnormalities);

- Haematological (eg low white blood count, leucopaenia);

- Metabolic (eg altered metabolic rate and glucose metabolism, impaired temperature regulation);

- Dermatological problems (eg dry scaly skin, discolouration, a fine layer of hair over the body);

- Endocrine (eg amenorrhoea, sexual impotence).

Cardiovascular complications are the most common, and are more likely to result in fatalities.[8] Congestive cardiac failure may occur as a terminal event, but also as a complication of refeeding. Osteoporosis (a condition that is characterized by decreasing bone mass which may cause bones to break more easily) is an early and irreversible consequence of severe weight loss. In long-term mortality studies, suicide is the commonest cause of death reported for anorexia nervosa.[9] The impact of the consequences of eating disorders on an individual's health and quality of life is illustrated in figures 1 and 2.[10] The consequences of anorexia nervosa are particularly severe, and all individuals with anorexia and bulimia nervosa suffer from psychological and physiological impairments, which have a serious impact on a sufferer's day-to-day functioning.

Figure 1: Assessments of ill-health in eating disordered patients at the Maudsley Hospital

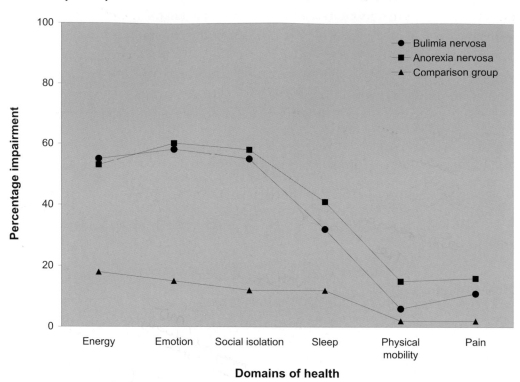

(Source: M Keilen, T Treasure, U Schmidt, J Treasure. Quality of life measures in eating disorders, angina, and transplant candidates, are they comparable? *Journal of the Royal Society of Medicine*;**87**:441-444, 1994)

Women who have a history of eating disorders may find that they have psychological difficulties during pregnancy. Women with bulimia who take laxatives can harm their foetuses and there can also be complications if a woman is severely restricting her diet while pregnant. In a 12.5 year follow-up study in Denmark, of the 50 anorexia nervosa sufferers who had children, the rate of prematurity among the offspring was twice the expected rate, and perinatal mortality (death rate from the 28th week of pregnancy to the end of the 1st week after birth) was six times the expected rate.[11] One premature child was visually impaired, 17% had poor growth in the first year of life, one child developed anorexia nervosa herself and died at the age of 15, one child was overweight and experiencing emotional and social problems, and one 5 year old had tritichollomania (compulsive hair pulling). A study of expectant mothers with bulimia nervosa[12] found that although by the third trimester (the last three months of pregnancy) 75% had stopped all bulimic behaviour, symptoms tended to return in the peurperium (the 6 weeks following childbirth). The incidence of foetal abnormality (including cleft palate and cleft lip), multiple pregnancies and obstetric complications was high. There is also a risk that underweight women may give birth to children who have an increased risk of coronary heart disease, non-insulin dependent diabetes and raised blood pressure.[13] In addition, evidence suggests that mothers with eating disorders have difficulties maintaining breastfeeding and make significantly fewer positive comments about food at mealtime observations with their offspring.[14] This could increase the risk that their own children will develop an eating disorder.

Figure 2: Assessments of functional impairments in eating disordered patients at the Maudsley Hospital

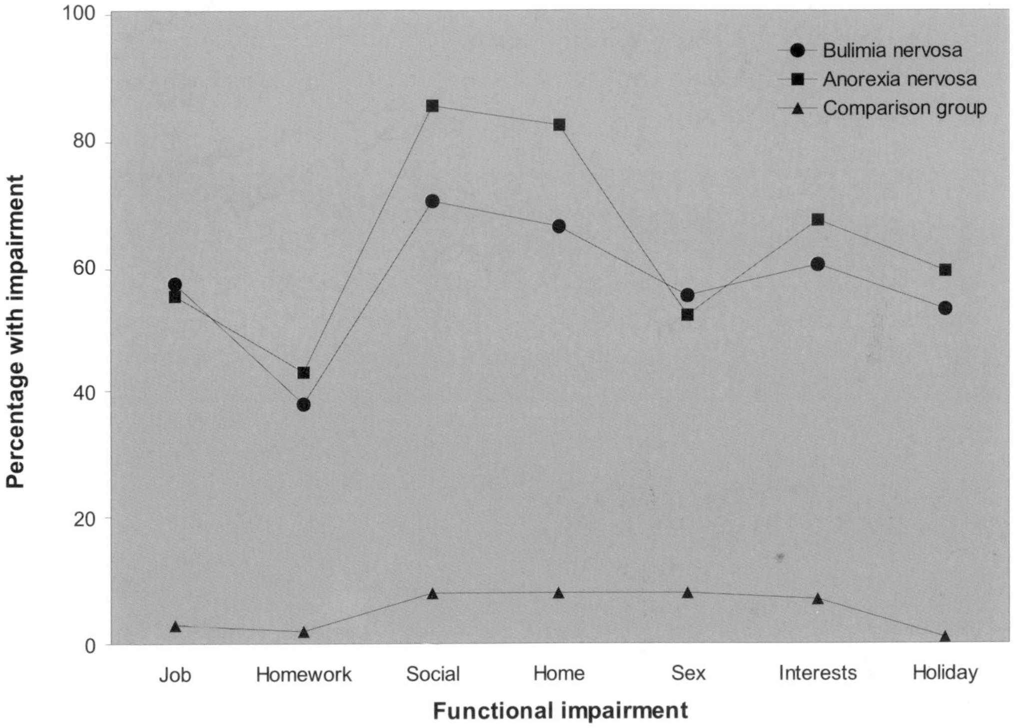

(Source: M Keilen, T Treasure, U Schmidt, J Treasure. Quality of life measures in eating disorders, angina, and transplant candidates, are they comparable? *Journal of the Royal Society of Medicine*;**87**:441-444, 1994)

Anorexia nervosa affects 1-2% of the UK female population between the ages of fifteen and thirty. Of these, between 6-10% die as a result of the illness.[15] Bulimia nervosa affects 1-5% of the female population.[15] The Royal College of Psychiatrists estimate that there are 60,000 eating disorder sufferers in the UK at any one time.[16] Ten percent of all individuals affected by eating disorders are men. It is estimated that an average GP, with a list of 2,000 patients, is likely to have one or two patients with anorexia nervosa and 18 patients with bulimia nervosa,[17] although in many cases they may not be detected. In a 4-15 year follow-up study of 460 eating disorder patients, it was found that there was a 600% increase in the mortality of anorexics when compared with the general population, and a 940% increase for bulimics,[18] although fewer people with bulimia appear to die as a direct result of their illness. The mortality risks of bulimia are less clearly defined in the literature. In a study of 103 patients with anorexia nervosa, followed up over 12 years, Herzog *et al*[19] found that 15% had died. Causes of death were within four areas: suicide, infection, gastro-intestinal complications and severe emaciation. The crude mortality rate for anorexia nervosa at 20 year follow-up may be as high as 15-20%.[2] In a meta-analyis of 42 published studies of the mortality rates for anorexia nervosa, it was found that the aggregate annual mortality rate associated with anorexia nervosa is more than 12 times higher than the annual death rate due to all causes of death for females 15-24 years old in the general population, and more than 200 times greater than the suicide rate in the general population.[20]

Summary Box

Eating disorders are a significant cause of mortality and morbidity in young people, particularly young women. Even if young people recover from an eating disorder, they may suffer long-term health problems as a result of their illness.

Aetiology — why do some people suffer from eating disorders?

The fundamental causes of anorexia and bulimia nervosa remain elusive. Theories abound, ranging from the biological and genetic to the environmental and behavioural. Modern thinking about the causation of anorexia nervosa considers factors that predispose, precipitate and perpetuate the disorder.[21] However, such terms are often employed in different contexts and with sociocultural factors in particular, it is often difficult to know how to label causal influences.

Di Nicola[22,23] outlines many different hypotheses of causation for anorexia nervosa, including the biomedical hypothesis which looks for an exclusive biological cause (eg primary hypothalamic dysfunction, the area of the brain in which the nervous and hormonal systems of the body interact); mood disorder hypothesis which considers eating disorders as primarily affective disorders; developmental psychobiological hypothesis which considers the role of pivotal triggering events during significant life changes (eg puberty); family and family systems hypothesis which consider the role of family conflict and the way that family units function; the feminist hypothesis which considers anorexia nervosa as a protest or reaction to social definitions of femininity; and the sociocultural hypothesis which considers why anorexia nervosa is a culturally bound syndrome and the way in which culture acts as a cause by providing a blueprint for eating disorders. It is this latter set of sociocultural factors that we will focus on, mainly concentrating on how the media provide blueprints for contemporary eating disorders. However, a brief overview of the other contributing factors may be useful in 'setting the scene'.

Biology, genetics and environment

Possible physical causes or precipitants of eating disorders have been identified in certain cases, for example lesions on the lateral hypothalamus,[24] post-viral infection[25] and Lyme disease.[26] Nevertheless, it is difficult to account for all cases of eating disorders in this way, at least until more evidence is uncovered.

Recent research has focused on the possible genetic component, which may predispose individuals to anorexia nervosa. Such research is based on familial and twin studies. Anorexia nervosa is around eight times more common in female first-degree relatives of individuals with anorexia nervosa than in the general population. It has been suggested that this is due to an inherited genetic vulnerability to adverse stress reactions caused by increased serotonin activity.[27] Twin studies have found higher concordance rates for anorexia nervosa in identical twins (56%) than in fraternal twins (5%).[28] It is, therefore, likely that there may be some underlying biological traits involving central nervous system neurotransmitters that contribute to the pathogenesis of eating disorders. However, much of this current research also suggests that there is an *interaction* between sociocultural, biological and genetic factors. There is a complex interplay between genetics, family history and the environment, and it is difficult to establish how many risk factors are genetic, and how many are acquired during development.[29] For example, it has been recently suggested that child rearing patterns may be significant for the later onset of eating disorders. A recent study has indicated that high-concern parenting in infancy is associated with the later development of anorexia nervosa.[30] It seems apparent that eating disorders cannot be explained by genetic factors alone.[31] In a study of 2,163 female twins, Kendler *et al* [32] found that genetic factors appeared to account for around 55% of the variance in inherited liability to bulimia nervosa, with the following sociocultural issues being identified as significant additional risk factors:

- Birth after 1960;

- Low paternal care;

- History of wide weight fluctuation, dieting or frequent exercise;

- Slim ideal body image;

- Low self-esteem;

- External locus of control (ie not feeling in control of one's own life);

- High levels of neuroticism.

A significant co-morbidity was found between bulimia and anorexia nervosa, alcoholism, panic disorder, generalised anxiety disorder, phobia and major depression. Familial studies, however, do not prove that eating disorders solely have a genetic cause, as "although it is possible that a familial disorder may be entirely genetic, familial aggregation can clearly be caused by genetic effects, environmental effects, or a combination of genes and environments".[33] In many cases the patterns of family relationships may be significant for the onset and continuation of the disorder; for example, the family's preferred style of handling conflict and how development of personal autonomy within the family is encouraged.

Personal, sociocultural and behavioural factors

The following personal, sociocultural and behavioural factors influencing the development of eating disorders in young people have been identified:[34]

Personal factors

Developmental factors (eg age, gender, pubertal development);

Cognitive/affective factors (eg nutritional knowledge and attitudes);

Psychological factors (eg self-esteem, body image, drive for thinness, depression, anxiety).

Socio-environmental factors

Sociocultural norms (eg regarding thinness, eating, food preparation, roles of women);

Familial factors (eg communication, expectations, weight concerns, family meals);

Peer norms and behaviours (eg dieting behaviours, eating patterns, weight concerns, social pressure);

Food availability (eg type of food, amount of food).

Behavioural factors:

Eating behaviours (eg meal patterns, fast-food consumption, nutritional variety, bingeing);

Dieting and other weight management behaviours (eg dieting frequency, types of diets, purging behaviour);

Physical activity or lack thereof (eg TV viewing, sport involvement, daily activities);

Coping behaviours (eg with dieting failures, with life frustrations);

Specific skills (eg self-efficacy in resisting harmful social norms, skills in food preparation).

Clearly, many of these factors are interrelated, and can be significant as predisposing, precipitating or perpetuating factors in particular individuals and contribute to a multifactorial theory of causation. The conceptual framework in figure 3 illustrates the multifactorial nature of eating disorders and how individual and family risk factors interact with wider sociocultural factors such as the pressure to be thin and beautiful.

Figure 3: Conceptual framework for development of eating disorders

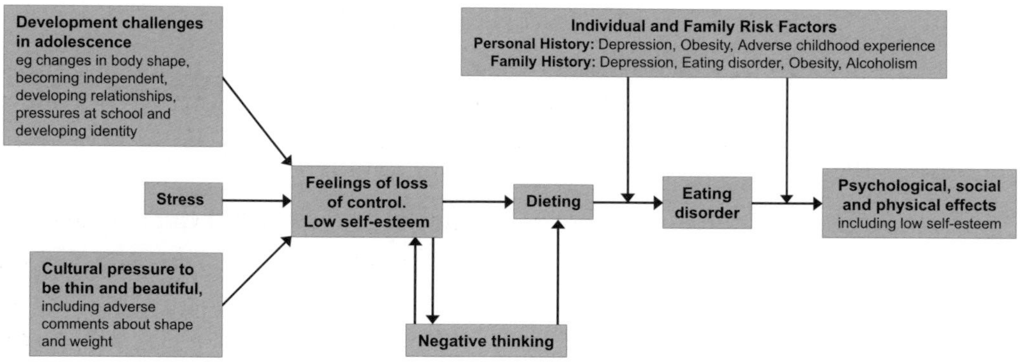

(Adapted from Stewart A. Experience with a school-based eating disorders prevention programme. In Walter Vandereycken and Greta Noordenbos. *The Prevention of Eating Disorders*. Athlone Press:Saffron Walden, 1998)

It may be useful to apply the concept of 'triggers' to eating disorders, when considering the impact of the media. Smolak and Levine[35] define triggers as "internal or external events or changes that initiate the questioning of existing psychological structures. Internal triggers include psychological and physical changes; external triggers may relate to role expectations". The media, for example, can be considered an external trigger which relays information about role expectations and appearance, and may be a significant factor in perpetuating the culture of thinness in modern society. However, the term may imply a short term 'cause and effect' which belies the slow and gradual acculturation of media values.

It is generally recognised that while there are many varied causes of eating disorders, society's aesthetic preference for thinness in women, for example, is a significant factor in the aetiology of eating disorders. It has been suggested that "anything that leads a woman to feel less secure and to value herself less may tip the balance towards things going wrong".[5] Young women face many confusing choices in today's society, relating to careers and relationships, and apparently many still feel that despite academic and career success, their personal value is still based on physical attractiveness to men. Having the 'right' body shape and size is widely valued as important to the goal of obtaining a partner. It is therefore potentially significant that young women are often presented with unobtainable images of bodily perfection by the media, and representations which may be particularly influential during adolescence — at a time when women can feel particularly insecure about their bodies and their potential attractiveness to members of the opposite sex. Adolescence and later teenage years are also periods where women can suffer from academic stress, peer pressure and insecurity about life goals, and choices which may produce eating disordered behaviour in vulnerable individuals ('vulnerable' may mean genetically predisposed, or individuals in a high risk environment, for example, in a highly achievement oriented family with perfectionist values, or with a strong interest in an activity like ballet which requires certain standards of body shape). The current emphasis given to the desirability of a slim body shape in Western society may play a major role in conditioning the preoccupations and behaviour of eating disorder sufferers.[36]

There are many different theoretical perspectives which can be used to illustrate sociocultural influences on eating disorders. One feminist perspective on eating disorders is that worrying about appearance is a 'normal' condition of contemporary femininity, and that the concentration on health and fitness (as dieting) for young women may be a way to provide the individual with some kind of control in a world that is hostile to feminine success and presence in the public sphere. It has also been pointed out that the beauty industry has commercialised women's liberation so that certain products are associated with independence and success.[37] The beauty industry has increasingly equated health with beauty, and fitness with sexuality, and have set up standards of perfection that were cast as unattainable, yet somehow within reach if only the right product was purchased. The perfect female body in the fashion and beauty industry is equated with a body that most closely resembles a man's, with few curves or excess fat. Another alternative psychoanalytic perspective focuses on the development of female sexuality and the role that anger, trauma and family conflict play in the development of personal identity. This report will take a more empirical approach and will not further examine the cultural studies perspective on eating disorders. However, it is important to recognise that alternative theoretical perspectives on eating disorders exist.

Dieting as a risk factor

There is a significant problem of increasing obesity levels in Western industrialised culture. In the UK, 17% of men and 20% of women are currently obese and over half of the adult population is overweight. If current trends continue, more than one quarter of British adults will be obese by the year 2010. It is not within the remit of this report to address the issues related to the media and obesity. However, it is necessary to examine issues related to dieting, and their impact on body perception and eating disorders. Fear of the social stigma attached to 'fatness' is one which may encourage many clinically underweight women to embark upon a programme of 'dieting', mistakenly believing that they are overweight. People who are perceived to be overweight are often the subject of ridicule and may be discriminated against in particular areas of life.[38] Many young women may enter into the 'culture of dieting', as being thin has many positive social connotations within our society, and models and actresses are admired for their thin body shapes.

The body mass index (BMI) is a convenient index of weight used by health professionals, it is calculated as weight/height^2 (in kgm^{-2}). Body Mass Index is generally graded as follows:

Grade III   BMI>40 kgm^{-2} — Gross Obesity

Grade II   BMI 30-39.9 kgm^{-2} — Obesity

Grade I   BMI 25-29.9 kgm^{-2} — Overweight

Grade O   BMI 20-24.9 kgm^{-2} — Acceptable[39]

Figure 4: BMI upper percentiles, British boys and girls

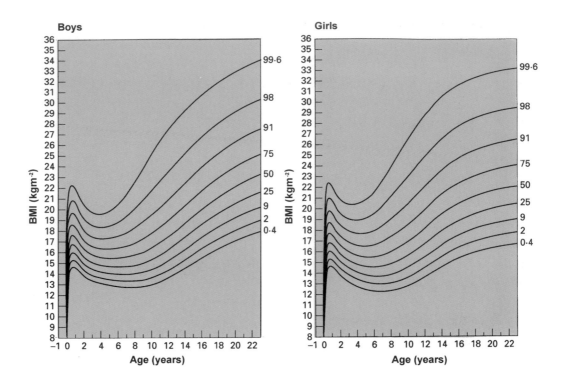

(Source: TJ Cole, JV Freeman, MA Preece. Body mass index reference curves for the UK, 1990. *Archives of Disease and Childhood*,1995;**73**:25-9)

The waist circumference or waist/hip ratio should also be included in the diagnosis of eating disorders, and allowances made for individual bone structures. For children, there are no acturial data on which to base cut-off points for obesity. However, it has been recommended that the upper percentiles of BMI references for British girls and boys can be used (see figure 4). Increasing levels of obesity may result in young people having a low self-image and a problematic relationship to food. Some young people may 'diet' without seeking appropriate medical guidance. The 'gap' between the thin ideal portrayed in the media and the reality of increasing obesity may further accentuate the child's perception that they are outside an acceptable social 'norm' and may result in a desire to lose weight dramatically. For adolescents and children, who are still in a critical phase of growth, dieting is a particularly hazardous practice — retarding normal growth and placing them at risk of developing an eating disorder.

Adolescent women entering the anorexia nervosa range of weights, can be identified using table 1[39]:

Table 1: Too thin: entering anorexia™ nervosa range*

Height without shoes (m)	Weight (kg)
1.45	38
1.48	39.5
1.50	40.5
1.52	41.5
1.54	42.5
1.56	44
1.58	45
1.60	46
1.62	47
1.64	48.5
1.66	49.5
1.68	50.5
1.70	52
1.72	53

*Body mass index of 18 kgm^{-2}

(Source: AS Trusswell. *ABC of Nutrition*. BMJ Books: London, 1999)

Although eating disorders should not be considered as just disorders of dieting, excessive dieting behaviour and other inappropriate weight loss practices are a central diagnostic feature. Dieting and dietary restraint is a necessary, but not sufficient, condition for eating disorders.[40] It is, however, a key risk factor, and dieting is a highly prevalent phenomenon in the most eating disorder-prone population of female adolescents and young adults. In a recent study carried out in Australia,[41] it was suggested that dieting is the most important predictor of new eating disorders. Of the 888 subjects studied, those who dieted at a severe level were 18 times more likely to develop an eating disorder than those who did not diet, and female subjects who dieted at a moderate level were five times more likely to develop an eating disorder than those who did not. An earlier study of schoolgirls in the UK concluded that the relative risk of a dieter being diagnosed with an eating disorder twelve months later, was eight times that of non-dieters.[42] These results indicate that for many young women the first step to an eating disorder is in trying to reduce body weight by dieting. Hsu[2] suggests that "adolescent dieting provides the entree into an eating disorder if such dieting is intensified by adolescent turmoil, low self and body concept, and poor identity formation".[2] Dieting, therefore, may not be the cause of eating disorders, but in many cases is the precipitant.[43, 44] It can be a particularly significant risk factor during puberty, when the percentage of fat on a young woman's body increases and there is heightened awareness of body image and physical attractiveness.[43] This conflict may be resolved by dieting, thus linking food with body image and self-esteem (and arguably, in some cases, a rejection of adulthood).

There should be increased awareness of the health risks for young women associated with being underweight and dieting, such as anaemia,[45] osteoporosis, early menopause and heart disease[46] and the risk of developing an eating disorder which could be fatal. In particular, there are serious physical consequences associated with dieting in younger age groups, as dieting in pre-adolescents may even further increase the risk of eating disorders.[44] In a recent UK study it was found that 93% of young women dieters failed to achieve the dietary requirements for iron intake.[47] The dieting group also failed to achieve an adequate intake of calcium, zinc and selenium.

Theoretically, dieting behaviour can be considered as an attempt to correct the disparity between our own body image and an idealised image. The media is a direct cultural source of our ideals. Research has shown that a large proportion of young women are dissatisfied with their body size and shape, and that dieting is on the increase amongst adolescent females.[48] In the Department of Health's Survey of Young People 1995-1997, 34% of young women aged 16-24 felt that they were too heavy, and only 5% felt that they were underweight.[48] Worryingly, even younger women are succumbing to the pressure to diet. In 1993 a study of 3,175 students in the US between the ages of 9 and 13 found that 40% of the respondents reported feeling fat or wishing to lose weight.[49] The link between our own body image and eating disorders becomes critical if current idealised body images are characterised by a degree of thinness which is unobtainable/ unachievable by most dieters.

Many young people at a nutritionally vulnerable period of life will skip breakfast,[50] and refuse regular family meals in favour of snacking or eating at fast food restaurants. This may lead to disordered eating patterns associated with increased morbidity and mortality.[51] Policy initiatives such as the provision of school breakfast clubs[13] may encourage children to view eating as a social activity to be enjoyed, and encourage positive associations with food.

It is apparent that we need to ask what leads some dieters to develop a full blown eating disorder whilst some young dieters do not? Other factors apart from media pressure to diet (eg environmental, psychological and genetic) may ultimately determine individual susceptibility to the clinical condition. For example, one research study has suggested dieting behaviour may be suspected for being potentially the first step in the downward spiral of a pursuit of thinness, if it is coupled with particular interpersonal problems, accentuated weight sensitivity, family conflicts, stress and fear of failure, and perfectionist tendencies.[52] However, this does not diminish the aetiological role of media imagery as a risk factor in eating disorders.

Summary Box

- Eating disorders are caused by a complex interplay between genetics, family history and the cultural environment.

- Social factors implicated in the development of eating disorders include sociocultural norms regarding thinness, eating, food preparation and roles of women.

- The media provide particular examples of role expectations and images of beauty which may influence young people's perceptions of acceptable body image.

- Obesity is an increasing problem in the UK, with adverse consequences for health. However, the considerable health risks for women associated with being underweight are less well publicised.

- Dieting is an important precipitant factor in the development of eating disorders. Young women are dieting at an increasingly young age, and expressing dissatisfaction with their body shapes.

- Many young people do not eat regular family meals and may not have positive associations with food. This may place them at risk of developing an eating disorder.

Eating problems in modern society

The medical literature indicates that eating disorders have become more prevalent in the latter half of the 20th century, although it should be borne in mind that increased awareness of the problem could have led to increased diagnosis. Two questions need to be asked: (1) Why do such disorders predominantly affect young women? and (2) Why did they become more common in the latter half of the 20th century? In assessing the reasons for this, it is useful to consider possible environmental factors that could be contributing to the predominance of eating disorders in contemporary Western industrialised cultures.

A review of the cultural and historical accounts of anorexia nervosa indicate that this disorder is found primarily in Westernised societies, particularly during periods of relative affluence and greater social opportunities for women. It has been suggested that anorexia nervosa is a culture-bound syndrome "in which the signs and symptoms of a disorder reflect psychosocial pressures or mores of certain cultures".[53]

Jules Bemporad's historical analysis[53] found that in the early history of Roman times and the Dark Ages there were few examples of wilful self-starvation, but those that did occur often had religious motivation. During the 13th-17th centuries there were many cases of wilful self-starvation related to holy fasting. He concluded that "the frequency and forms of anorexia during the Renaissance may be explained partially by the marked changes in everyday life and in cultural values initiated by the relative wealth and sophistication associated with the period of history". Anorexia nervosa was only first described as a psychiatric condition and distinguished from other forms of starvation in the 19th century. The careful comprehensive delineation of signs and symptoms was exemplified by Lasegue (1873)[54] and Gull (1874),[55] who presented a complete medical description of anorexia nervosa. In the past few decades there has been an increased incidence of this disorder, a greater emphasis on fear of fatness, and the emergence of bulimia nervosa as a new disorder (bulimia nervosa was defined by Gerald Russell in 1979).[56]

Bemporad's analysis of eating disorders outlines a form of behaviour that flourished at certain periods of history, receded in others, and became a far greater problem in the latter part of the 20th century than ever before. Examination of clinical case registers have indicated a rise in the number of cases of eating disorders, for example:

- New cases of anorexia nervosa in one area of New York doubled from the period 1960-1967 to 1970-1976.[57]

- An examination of the psychiatric case notes in Aberdeen in the period 1965-1982 showed a highly significant increase in cases of anorexia and bulimia nervosa.[58]

- The incidence of eating disorders in Spain has been increasing by 15% a year, and a mulitidisciplinary working party was established by the Spanish Health Ministry in April 1999 to investigate the problem.[59]

Ethnicity

A cross-cultural analysis also indicates that eating disorders in part may be culturally or environmentally determined. The literature indicates that fewer Asian and black women than white women suffer eating disorders. The incidence among all ethnic minorities judged from clinical case registers is lower than that of whites.[60] In a recent study at the Leicestershire Eating Disorders Service within a catchment area with a large Asian population, twenty one eating disordered Asians were seen in 10 years — this was a rate at one-fourth of the white population.[61]

Although it may be that people from ethnic minorities are less likely to be diagnosed with eating disorders, and referred to appropriate services, it would appear that the disorders are less prevalent in non-whites. In an analysis of black women and eating disorders in the US, Striegel-Moore and Smolak[62] concluded that black women's "gender roles, compared to those of white women, seem less shaped by an emphasis on outward appearance and more determined by pride in self and community". Wider social support networks, therefore, may offer protection against low self-esteem and poor body image. It has been suggested that white women chose a significantly thinner ideal body size, and that there is far less emphasis on thinness in black culture — black men, for example, apparently express more willingness to date 'larger-than-ideal' women.[63] It would appear that external factors to the media are helping certain sectors of the population resist pressure to conform to particular body shapes.

There have only been very few cases of anorexia nervosa reported from developing countries. There are higher rates amongst immigrants to Western society, and rising frequency amongst ethnic minority populations who have been raised in Western industrialised culture.[2] In one study of Kenyan immigrants to Britain, it was found that Kenyan women tended to rate larger female figures more favourably than Caucasian British women, while Kenyan British women who had been in the UK for at least four years, were more similar to the Caucasian British women in their perceptions of body size.[64] Eating disorders are increasingly prevalent in Singapore,[65] and other countries that have followed the Western model of socio-economic development. It therefore seems wise to assume that factors associated with Western culture are influencing these women.

Men

Men comprise 10% of eating disorder sufferers,[4] but many more may find it hard to recognise the symptoms or seek appropriate help. Men, in particular, may not have their symptoms recognised at an early stage and be referred to specialist services and may, therefore, suffer poor health outcomes.[66] Most of the published literature discusses the aetiology of anorexia nervosa as it applies to women, and may sometimes be gender specific (eg some of the psychoanalytic arguments that state that females may develop anorexia nervosa when they are struggling to create a separate identity from their mothers). The problem remains, when researching eating disorders, that very little published work relates specifically to males. However, this reflects the fact that they comprise a small percentage of eating disorder sufferers.

In one study, Margo[66] suggested that the two most important factors for developing eating disorders in both men and women were a family history of psychiatric illness and a deviation from the perceived normal body shape. This manifested itself as dissatisfaction with small stature in males and large stature in females. It is claimed that "...the small male, like the large or very tall female, risks becoming preoccupied about his size and deviation from what he considers a desirable physique". In another study[67] the following aetiological factors of eating disorders in men were cited — obsessional personality, skewed parental relationships, self-consciousness about being overweight and, importantly, an apprehension of the threat of manhood, with particular reference to the heterosexual role.

If the media play a role in triggering eating disorders, then we would expect that as men become more preoccupied with their looks and are increasingly targeted by advertisers (for example, in new men's magazines) they may develop a higher incidence of eating disorders.[68] It has been suggested that men who are homosexual, for example, show greater tendencies toward eating disorders, as their culture places greater emphasis on bodily perfection and physical appearance.[69] Young men are also facing uncertainty and confusion about their changing role in society. This may be reflected in the fact that the suicide rate for young males has more than doubled from 6.9 per 100,000 of the population in 1971, to 16.4 per 100,000 of the population in 1997.[70] New ways of increasing self-esteem in young men that also reflect the changing nature of the traditional female roles and the family, must be considered. However, it may still be the case that for the majority of men, body insecurity will manifest itself in other behaviours; for example, obsessive use of the gymnasium or the use of steroids to increase musculature or enhance body mass.[46] In a recent series of interviews with body builders using anabolic steroids, all the men interviewed cited pressure from images in body building magazines, and images from film and television, as being influential in their decision to take steroids.[46] It should, however, be remembered that social reality is complex, and individuals with poor body image may seek out particular forms of media consumption.

A recent study in the US[71] which analysed survey data obtained from 9,118 adolescents from the 8th, 9th and 11th grade, found that disordered eating over the previous week was reported by 7.4% of the girls and 3.1% of the boys. It was found that girls in the highest body mass index (BMI) categories were at greatest risk for disordered eating behaviours, while boys in the lowest BMI category were at greatest risk for steroid use. This evidence reflects the view that when young boys report dissatisfaction with their weight it is often due to the desire to be heavier, whereas girls want to be thinner.[3,48,72] As dieting is often the precursor to developing an eating disorder,[2] the cultural ideal for men to be larger and stronger may offer men protection from developing an eating disorder on the same scale as women, unless they have additional sociocultural risk factors such as having been previously overweight and been subject to criticism or teasing, have gender role confusion or are engaged in a sport where weight loss is required[73] (for example, rowing or horse racing). Significantly, it has been estimated that 25% of men diet at some point in their lives, compared to 95% of women.[46]

Although anorexia and bulimia nervosa mainly affect young women by a ratio of 10:1, many of the arguments in this report apply equally to males with eating disorders. Developing self-esteem and healthy attitudes towards food, are goals that we should try to achieve for all of our young people, male and female.

Eating disorders — a culturally bound phenomenon

Anorexia nervosa is a culturally bound phenomenon largely associated with Western industrialised societies. It has been suggested that the following characteristics of Western industrialised societies have contributed to the prevalence of the disease in these societies:

- a changing female role, in which women find themselves struggling to strike a balance between new ideals of achievement and traditional female role expectations;

- a preoccupation with appearance and body image that is associated with the rise of mass fashion and consumerism; and

- a culturally pervasive preoccupation with weight control and obesity.[74]

In societies that do not value thinness, eating disorders are very rare.[75] The media obviously have a role in perpetuating the culture of thinness in contemporary Western societies, as they are major sources of our ideas about fashion and desirable body image. They are particularly influential in childhood and early adolescence where the association with branded goods and external appearance are particularly important sources of identity, and belonging to a peer group. The use of thin models to advertise glamorous products contrasts sharply with the actual body size of the majority of women in Western industrialised societies (for a discussion of this discrepancy between media images and actual female body size see page 33). It has been suggested that the media culture has contributed to a situation in which "most women can feel good about themselves only in a state of permanent semi-starvation".[76] In general, there is a negative cultural attitude to being overweight or obese — overweight people are mainly portrayed as figures of ridicule by the media, and successful female celebrities find that their weight loss or weight gain is the main focus of media attention and speculation.

Summary Box

- Eating disorders became more prevalent in Western industrialised countries in the latter part of the 20th century.

- Fewer Asian and black women apparently suffer from eating disorders, although there are higher rates amongst immigrants to Western society and ethnic minority populations raised in Western industrialised cultures, or those following a Western model of development.

- Eating disorders predominantly effect young women. However, evidence from studies of men with eating disorders also suggest that perceived body image measured against a societal 'norm' is a crucial factor in the onset of the illness.

- Although certain biological predispositions (which may in part be genetically determined) may contribute to the onset of eating disorders in an individual, historical and cross-cultural evidence suggests that the development of eating disorders is significantly influenced by particular aspects of modern society.

- It is important that we consider the possible social influences that contribute to the onset of eating disorders, and examine reasons why eating disorders predominantly affect young women living in Western industrialised cultures.

Role of the media

It would appear that one of the main reasons why anorexia nervosa and bulimia nervosa are culturally-bound syndromes is that they depend on the culture of thinness pervading those nations where disorders are prevalent. One of the most important means of generating and maintaining the culture of thinness are those adopted purposely or accidentally through the media and advertising. The following section will look at some of the possible mechanisms of influence and their effects.

The media are an important component of everyday life in Western society. By 1995, 99% of the UK population owned a television set.[77] Watching television is the most popular home-based activity in the UK.[78] On average people in the UK spend 25 hours a week watching television, with women watching more television than men.[78] In 1997-98, 61% of men and 52% of women read a national daily newspaper.[78] Readership of magazines by girls aged 7-14 is quite high amongst the target audience, with 34% of the 7-10 age group reading the most popular magazine *Girl Talk*, and 47% of the 11-14 age group reading the magazine *Sugar*.[78] The most popular magazines for adults are connected to television viewing. Television remains the most popular form of mass media, and most of us are regularly exposed to its content.

Children, food and the media

It has been estimated that children in the US view around 20,000 TV commercials a year.[79] Although television in the UK is not as heavily commercialised, the introduction of cable and satellite television into more homes will undoubtedly increase the exposure of children to television advertising, as these channels tend to rely more heavily on some forms of marketing for their revenue. One recent UK study found that in homes with cable and satellite facilities, children increased their viewing by 90 minutes a week between 1992 and 1995.[80]

Battle and Brownwell[81], have argued that the media contribute to a 'toxic environment' in which eating disorders may be more likely to occur. They illustrate this by referring to the damaging paradox of modern society that "while an extremely lean, contoured, and sculpted body is the ideal, and that repeated, compelling exposure to this unrealistic ideal is the norm, the environment provides access to, and encourages consumption of a diet that is high in fat and calories".[81] Children and young people who are regularly exposed to the media, receive a confusing message, as thin models and actors are often employed to advertise high calorie soft drinks or fast food. Unhealthy attitudes towards food, body shape and exercise may be nurtured in this 'toxic environment'. The images of slim models on television is a stark contrast to the body size and shape of most children and young women, who are becoming increasingly heavier. The association of thinness with success and acceptance is one that may have long-lasting effects on body image and self-esteem.

Theories of media influence

In order to understand the role of the media, it is useful to briefly consider some of the research that has been conducted on the effects of the media on behaviour. The mass media have been defined by Levine and Smolak[82] in their analysis of media influences on eating disorders as:

"...publicly supported institutions and forms of communications that generate messages designed for a very large, very heterogenous, and essentially anonymous audience...the messages serve many purposes, including entertainment, education, government and, of course, engagement of huge groups of people so that advertisers can sell them products. Children, adolescents, and adults interact with a wide variety of mass media, including television, music delivered by compact discs and radio, and telecommunications available through personal computers."

They consider that types of mass media which may be especially relevant to eating disorders include fashion magazines, television and self-help weight-loss books.

The media in Western industrialised countries are such an important component in the majority of people's everyday lives that they can be seen as permeating the culture of these societies. The effect that the media have on our behaviour is a subject of continuous debate. In the 1920s-1930s, an approach to the media known as 'Mass Society Theory' argued that the media are powerful forces which can exploit and manipulate individuals (known as the 'hypodermic' approach as it supposed that the media 'injected' certain values into its audience). Social psychological research into media effects in the 1940s-60s, however, indicated that the audience often selected and filtered information and rejected messages which were not consonant with existing beliefs or attitudes.[83] For example, in a series of film evaluation studies of training films for US soldiers in the 1940s, it was found that individual differences led to selective perception, interpretation and change of opinion, and that membership of certain social categories — eg educational attainment — could often predict a particular response.[84] In later studies on communication and persuasion it was found that people who valued their membership of particular social groups were least affected by communications that advocated positions contrary to the norms of the group. Individual personality factors were also examined, and it was discovered that persons who have low self-esteem were easily influenced.[84]

The influence of the media on behaviour is much more complicated than stimulus and response, and we need to consider the interaction between the types of media messages transmitted and the kinds of audience receiving the messages. Studies of the effects of television violence on behaviour have indicated that "television's most profound influences may be indirect."[84]

During the 1960s, research into media effects was criticised for taking a short-term view of its audience, which did not look at the long-term effects of exposure to certain images and values. In the 1980s a 'postmodern' approach was increasingly taken to media texts, considering that media images have become a primary sources for shaping personal identity and social reality.[83] In a media saturated culture, the argument that long-term exposure can help shape the world views of particular sections of the audience, is one that merits consideration. However, the *extent* to which the media contribute to personal identity remains unclear, and is subject to continuing academic debate. There is more consensus that the media are instrumental in creating and reinforcing particular beliefs and opinions. The media do not, by their very definition, provide pure experience of the world, but channel our experience of it in particular ways. A 1982 report[85] on television and behaviour concluded that:

"Almost all evidence testifies to television's role as a formidable educator whose effects are both persuasive and cumulative. Television can no longer be considered as a casual part of daily life, as an electronic toy. Research findings have long since destroyed the illusion that television is merely innocuous entertainment. While the learning it provides is mainly incidental rather than direct and formal, it is a significant part of the total acculturation process."

Rather than focusing on exposure to one TV advertisement or one particular model, the cumulative long-term effects of the media on young people's behaviour should be considered. The effects of the media are diffused in society, to the extent that it is difficult to single out particular examples of it directly influencing behaviour. The media are undoubtedly one of the most powerful cultural influences that young people in Western cultures are exposed to, and can often define parameters of normative behaviour. However, it is particularly important not to think of media influence in a completely negative framework. The 1982 report on television and behaviour also concluded that TV content can produce prosocial behaviour.

Although this report has mainly focussed on empirical research into media effects, there are many different perspectives on the mechanisms of media influence. As Lowery and DeFleur conclude in their analysis of media research

"…it is difficult to locate eternal verities about the process of mass communication using the strategies of science while searching through the shifting sands of social, cultural and technological change."[84] We must remember the temporal nature of media content, technologies and consumption, and recognise that this is a subject which is constantly in a state of flux. New interactive media technologies, for example, may further complicate the literature on media effects, and it may be increasingly possible to influence the direction and content of media programming.

There is a need to distinguish between different media content. For example, the media's influence may be particularly strong when 'advertising' is employed, as advertising is specifically designed to influence behaviour. Although we should avoid falling into the 'Mass Society Theory' trap of thinking that advertisements are a form of 'brainwashing', the effects, particularly on children, are likely to be more persuasive than those of other forms of media,[86] and advertisers are likely to use images of thin women more often than other body types. On an annual basis, children spend more time in front of the TV than they do at school. Therefore it has been concluded that "television represents a major source of information about the world, how people act, what people eat, and how they look".[87] Television advertising, in particular, may generate social comparison in some circumstances.[88] However, all research on 'media effects' needs to consider the contextual complexities involved in receiving media messages: the media do not 'brainwash' people, but receive different levels of attention and interpretation by individuals with different motivations, personalities, immediate situations and sociocultural contexts, who bring different information processing strategies to the task.[89] The media are not monolithic, and do not effect everybody in the same way. They also provide positive contributions to people's lives as major sources of enjoyment, education and conversation, which should not be forgotten when we address some of the possible negative aspects of their role in contemporary society.

Studies of media influence on perceptions of body shape and size

Some studies have specifically looked at the media's influence on eating disorders. A selection of the type of research that has been conducted is summarised below.

Media content

It is estimated that at least 50% of adolescent girls regularly read fashion and beauty related magazines[82] and these are read more frequently by girls aged 11-15. Levine and Smolak[82] state that this high level of involvement in teenage magazines coincides with a peak level of exposure to television, which also emphasises the importance of appearance and slenderness to females, at a time when the young female's self-perception is in decline and where she may compare herself to others to a greater degree. Schoolgirls may find themselves in a 'subculture of dieting', reflecting the intersection of consistent messages from family, peers and the media regarding acceptable body size and shape.[90]

Content analyses of women's magazines have consistently found that articles concentrate on beauty and diet, and have outlined the declining curvaceousness of models used for fashion magazines (see for example, Silverstein et al[91] Andersen and DiDomenico[92]). Guillen and Barr[93] found that in their analysis of women's magazines over the period 1970-1990, the numbers of articles dedicated to nutrition did not increase over the years, but those on fitness did. The articles on nutrition and fitness emphasised body shape and appearance and the thin body shape ideal, and the primary reasons presented for following a nutrition or fitness plan, were to lose weight or become more attractive.

Research has also found that most female characters on television are thinner than average women. In 1980, a study of *Playboy* magazines during the period 1959-1978 found that there was a 10% decrease in weight for height over the models used during this 20 year period. More significantly, this represented a much greater discrepancy between the magazine images and the actual size of women in society as a whole, as women became heavier during that period.[94] In a similar study it was found that the mean bust-to-waist ratio of 15 actresses appearing for the first time in 1940-1959 was 1.34, while the ratio for actresses appearing for the first time in 1960-1979 was 1.22.[91] It has been estimated that models and actresses in the 1990s have 10%-15% body fat — the average body fat for a healthy woman is 22-26%.[95] This kind of research, however, has been criticised for not considering the effects of exposure to this media content. To say that the number of thin women represented in the media has increased, and that women's magazines concentrate on issues surrounding beauty and diet, does not provide us with any information on how these images are received by the audience.

Effect of media content

Some experiments have been conducted which have attempted to combine content analyses with a questionnaire study or interview of young people in order to assess the impact of certain images or media values on young people's worldview. In a study of 94 adolescent women reporting what television programmes they had watched in the previous week, it was found that the amount of television watched did not correlate with body dissatisfaction and drive for thinness, but category of programme was significant. The women who were aged

15 years old, watched 3.2 hours of television a day, on average. Body dissatisfaction was significantly positively correlated with watching soap operas or serials, and movies. Drive for thinness was correlated with time spent watching music videos. Body satisfaction increased with watching sports.[96] It is difficult, however, to establish any causality between types of television programme watched and the development of an eating disorder, as young people who are dissatisfied with their bodies may seek out particular kinds of television viewing.[35]

In a study of 548 12th grade schoolgirls in the US,[97] 69% reported that magazine pictures influence their idea of the perfect body shape, and 47% reported wanting to lose weight because of pictures in magazines. There was a positive linear association between the frequency of reading women's magazines and the prevalence of having dieted to lose weight because of a magazine article, initiating an exercise programme because of a magazine article, wanting to lose weight because of pictures in magazines, and feeling that pictures in a magazine influence their idea of the perfect body shape. The authors from this study concluded that "...the print media aimed at young girls could serve a public health role by refraining from relying on models who are severely underweight and printing more articles on the benefits of physical activity."

Research conducted by Pinhas et al[98] found that women who viewed images of fashion models scored more highly on a scale designed to measure depression and anger, than they had before viewing the images. They also scored more highly than women who had viewed slides of neutral objects. Hamilton and Waller[99] describe the media as a 'negative reinforcer' of an overestimated body size in women with eating disorders. The study compared 24 eating disordered women and 24 women who did not have any signs of anorexia or bulimia nervosa. The women were shown two sets of photographs of women in fashion magazines and 20 photographs of neutral objects from a interior design magazine. The women looked at the photographs for 20 seconds, rated them for attractiveness, and then estimated their own body size. The women without eating disorders were not affected by the nature of the photographs, but eating disordered women were — they overestimated their body size more when they had seen the pictures of women than when they saw photographs of neutral objects. It is hard to draw any conclusions on the media's role in eating disorder aetiology from a study based on a small number of women in laboratory or survey conditions and longer term ethnographic research is needed to assess how the media is actually received and interpreted by women in everyday life.

Cross cultural evidence

Evidence from countries newly exposed to Western media culture provide useful indicators of its impact on cultural trends. Ann Becker, an anthropologist at Harvard Medical School who has been studying eating habits in Fiji since 1988, has identified an increase in eating disorders in Fiji since the arrival of television in 1995. In 1998, she conducted a survey of teenage girls in Fiji and found that 74% of them felt that they were too big or fat. This contrasts with the traditional Fijian preference for large builds for both sexes, and previous research which indicated that thinness was associated with social neglect and deprivation.[100] It would appear that Western ideals of beauty have led to a high percentage of adolescents dieting within the last decade. Similar research in the Cook Islands has shown that traditional Polynesian concepts of very large body sizes as healthy and attractive are no longer in evidence.[101] However, it is extremely difficult to prove that it has been exposure to the media images that has caused this change in the experience of adolescent Fijian girls and Polynesian women, rather than other factors associated with 'Westernisation.' Nevertheless, it would seem reasonable to assume that the arrival of television has played a significant part in the development of dieting behaviour within this culture.

Summary

These studies are a small selection of those that have attempted to assess the impact of media imagery on body image and the development of eating disorders. It is difficult to establish any causation between exposure to media imagery and low self-esteem and negative attitudes to the body, as many of these studies do not consider the effects of long-term exposure to media imagery, and are often based on small samples of women. A comprehensive review of the literature by Levine and Smolak[82] supports the notion that "there is a great deal of theorising and media criticism available, but far too little systematic research."[82] However, in reaching that conclusion, the authors suggest that the media may play a wider role in shaping our reactions to body size and quote from work conducted on body image by Tolman and Debold: "The image of the desirable women (sic) is posed as the model of success. She is a painfully familiar sight, appearing before us in the mass media and reflected in the expectations of others. There are few women who have not negotiatied some relationship with her."[102]

Women appear to worry about their weight more than any other possible health risk — for example in one study (figure 5),[78] women were found to perceive their weight as a greater risk to health than smoking or alcohol consumption. Men rated the threat from pollution, lack of exercise, and smoking above concerns about weight.

Figure 5: Adults' view of what is bad for their health: by gender, 1996

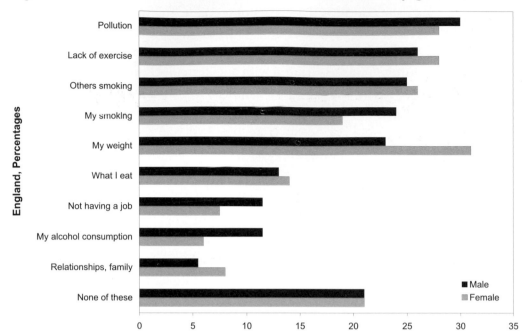

(Source: *Social Trends 29* Office for National Statistics Crown Copyright 1999)

Clearly, for women, weight is a major concern — the daily exposure to weight-related articles in newspapers, magazines and on television, and the thinness of role models in the fashion industry must undoubtedly contribute to feelings of insecurity and self-doubt about acceptable body image.

Summary Box

- The media are a significant and pervasive influence in modern society, and provide information about gender roles, fashion and acceptable body image which may be particularly influential on those young children and adolescents who are heavily exposed to its content.

- Advertising, in particular, may influence young people's perception of fashion, beauty and attitudes towards food.

- Some studies have attempted to illustrate the importance of the media on women's perception of body shape, although many studies are based on small samples of women and are unable to consider the long-term effects of media exposure on body image.

- Young women may compare themselves to extremely thin models, working in the fashion industry or advertising products, and perceive themselves as 'fat' in comparison, rather than healthy and attractive.

Media influence on body image and self-esteem

The evidence considered (eg Field *et al* 1999, Pinhas *et al* 1999, Hamilton and Waller 1991) suggests that the media have an important role in shaping women's image of themselves, and the ideal body shapes in society. The following section will examine the role of the media in encouraging a faulty perception of optimum body size in the large majority of women. These influences may induce a large proportion of adolescent girls and young women to adopt the practice of restrictive dieting, which may lead to adverse effects.

Body image is a key concept in understanding the influence of the media on a sense of personal identity, and has been defined as "the physical and cognitive representation of the body which underlies and includes attitudes of acceptance and rejection."[103] Clearly, body image is closely linked to self-esteem, and negative body image is a key aspect of eating disorders.[104] It has been claimed that media imagery may be particularly important in producing changes in the way the body is perceived and evaluated.[46] Myers and Biocca[105] have used the concept of 'the elastic body image' to examine this role. The media contribute to the socially represented ideal body by providing examples of 'attractive' women — ie models, actresses and pop stars — which provide a point of comparison for women to measure themselves against. It is suggested that women configure an 'internalised ideal body' by comparing their actual body shape against the socially represented ideal body. This results in a present body image, which is 'elastic' in the sense that at different times under different stresses and influences women can view their own bodies against these different reference points.

In recent years the socially represented ideal body has become increasingly thin, and much thinner than the average objective body shape of the population, putting pressure on women to view their bodies as fatter and heavier.[105] This has been illustrated by recent research on young women. In a study of 869 Australian schoolgirls aged 14-16 years it was found that two thirds of the total sample perceived themselves as fat, although only 16% were actually overweight, 87% of the total sample desired the thin 'ideal' body shape promoted by the media. One third of the females had used at least one of the extreme weight reduction practices within the previous month — crash dieting (22%), fasting (21%) and smoking (12%). The study concluded that motivating factors for disordered eating and unhealthy dieting behaviours amongst Australian adolescent girls were peer pressure, media pressure, and the perception that extreme dieting strategies were harmless.[106]

Myers and Biocca[105] conclude that messages of beauty and attractiveness in the media are a contributing factor to these body distortions. In another study which looked at the 'thin ideal' stereotypc's effect on body perception, results indicated that exposure to the 'thin ideal' produced depression, stress, guilt, shame, insecurity and body dissatisfaction in the women studied.[107]

Despite increasing acadcmic success and participation in public life, many young women appear to be suffering from a crisis of low self-esteem. A recent survey by the Flour Advisory Bureau[108] questioned 901 women aged 18-24 about their influences, sources of self-esteem, body image and eating habits. The survey found that:

- One in five young women diet all or most of the time because of the pressure they feel under to meet unrealistic expectations of physical perfection.

- Social and peer group pressure has left young women with distorted perceptions of what is a healthy weight, and the belief that unless they have waif-like figures they will be turned down for jobs and rejected by men.

- Graduate career women are more likely to feel guilty about eating than any other group.

When asked how they feel compared to the pictures of young women portrayed by the media, almost half identified the pictures with the description that made them feel 'inadequate'. The messages given to young women are often conflicting.[109] Women are expected to be thin, attractive, successful in the workplace, ambitious and financially independent, while maintaining their traditional roles as nurturing, maternal, warm, supportive wives, homemakers and mothers.[110] Women who cannot reconcile these roles may seek the security of controlling weight to bolster fragile self-esteem, or a displacement activity to avoid making difficult life decisions.

One study has indicated the importance of developing self-esteem in young women, as a possible preventative measure for eating disorders.[111] The study assessed self-esteem in 594 schoolgirls aged 11-12 years, and reassessed 400 of the girls at age 15-16, and asked them to complete a questionnaire examining eating disorders and psychological problems (the other 194 had either changed schools or their parents had refused participation in the follow-up). Those in the lowest self-esteem range were about eight times more at risk of developing a high Eating Attitudes Test score (used to assess eating disorders) than those in the highest self-esteem range. The results indicated that girls with low self-esteem at age 11-12 were at significantly greater risk of developing severe signs of eating disorders and other psychological problems at age 15-16. The study also indicated that eating problems and disorders overlap with other psychological stresses, such as the stress of taking GCSE exams. Self-esteem is considered to be a reflection of a variety of influences including genetic endowment, educational achievement, quality of family life and social conditions. Parental and peer influence to diet can significantly predict dietary restraint.[40] Comments about weight in the family (for example, by grandparents) may act as a precipitant factor for the onset of eating disorders, and may lower self-esteem and link thinness to being successful or loved. In one study[90] two strong correlates for the drive for thinness and disturbed patterns of eating were identified: reading magazines that contain information and ideas about an attractive body shape and about weight management, and weight/shape-related teasing and criticism by the family. Low self-esteem may increase the likelihood of acceptance of media messages, and those messages may further damage self-esteem by providing examples of unrealistic body shapes as 'ideal'.

It has been suggested that women in Western culture exhibit a 'normative discontent' with their bodies and that efforts to prevent eating disorders could potentially benefit many more individuals than those with a diagnosed disorder.[81] There are many indicators of this 'normative discontent' with the body in our culture.[46] The rise of cosmetic surgery, for example, is in many cases a useful indicator of low self-esteem and concern with physical appearance often rooted in adolescent identity conflicts[29] — although this may also merely reflect a rise in disposable income. Many women willingly risk physical discomfort and surgical procedures to obtain bodily perfection. In the US, women comprise 89% of people undergoing plastic surgery.[112] A study in the United States indicated that among women who wished to have the size of their breasts reduced, more than half of the cases were found to show symptoms of either anorexia or bulimia nervosa.[52] A recent study has concluded that smoking is associated with the pursuit of thinness in women with bulimia nervosa.[113] Many women also continue to smoke in the mistaken belief that it will keep them thin, and refuse to give up smoking for fear of weight gain.[114] Poor self-esteem and negative attitudes towards body shape appear to be widespread amongst young females in Western industrialised society.

Efforts to prevent eating disorders could, in addition, remove or reduce the 'normative discontent' that women in Western culture exhibit. For women without eating disorders, such measures might also lead to a decrease in potentially dangerous behaviours such as unnecessary cosmetic surgery and smoking, in order to improve body image.

In many of the case histories of eating disorders and in the descriptions of trigger causes for the onset of the disease, low self-esteem would appear to be a prevalent psychological precursor to the development of an eating disorder. The media may contribute to low self-esteem in young women by promoting slenderness as the path to social, sexual and occupational success. There is a cultural emphasis on the possibility, desirability and safety of personal transformation through fashion and dieting, and an open abhorrence of women who are perceived to be fat.[115] When young women were asked how they would most like to be described in a recent survey, most chose non-physical attributes like kind and caring, intelligent and confident, and yet when asked what men found most attractive in women, 55% responded that looks were the most attractive thing in a woman.[108] Only 1% said that men found intelligence the most attractive thing in a woman, 62% felt that looks would affect their chances of getting a boyfriend and 52% said it would affect their career prospects. It is clear that many young women feel that they are judged on their looks rather than their achievements.

Today's young woman is expected to strive for perfection in all spheres. Perfectionism is a strong risk factor for the development of an eating disorder. It has been suggested by social analyst Helen Wilkinson that young women today often feel pressurised by the opportunities to succeed and "through their problematic relationship to food are in retreat from them or are engaged in a complex and often subconscious process of self sabotage".[116] Many women have unhealthy and dysfunctional attitudes towards food, and even those who do not suffer from eating disorders exhibit signs of disordered eating, which may lead to restricted food intake or 'faddism'. Eating large meals can be seen as 'unfeminine' and women may feel cultural pressure to restrict food intake.[117]

Advertising control — ITC and ASA policies

The BMA is concerned about the use of very thin models to advertise products, and to model clothes for the fashion industry. The Independent Television Commission's (ITC) existing policy states that it is desirable to ensure that advertising for slimming products does not help stimulate unhealthy attitudes to eating and that such advertisements "must not suggest or imply that to be underweight is acceptable or desirable". Those giving testimonials must not appear to be underweight. However, this only covers slimming products as the ITC believes that there is not enough evidence to show that the use of underweight models in advertising can directly influence the onset of anorexia nervosa. A public censure was issued by the Advertising Standards Authority (ASA) in 1998 for an advert by a wristwatch manufacturer where it was considered that the use of a very thin model to advertise the product was irresponsible. However, there are still many examples of thin models being used in advertisements, and more particularly there are very few overweight, or normal sized women used to model clothes. The degree of thinness exhibited by the models chosen to promote products is often both unachievable and also biologically inappropriate, and provides unhelpful role models for young women.

Positive media influence

Anorexia and bulimia nervosa are serious psychological illnesses, which require considerable medical intervention and may be, in part, genetically determined. However, a public health model of illness can be employed if we consider that environmental factors can influence the onset and course of the illness, and that we can take certain steps to reduce risk factors for vulnerable individuals.

Although the media may play a significant — if hard to quantify — role in the aetiology of eating disorders, it should be one of the more controllable factors that we can influence. It is important to realise that the media do not influence women's self-esteem in an exclusively negative direction. The media can have a constructive and helpful role in encouraging young women to feel confident about themselves and their role in society, and can play a crucial role in encouraging healthy eating habits and relationships to food.

The media play a significant role to health promotion. In a study of women aged 16-24, the Health Education Authority[118] has found that teenage and women's magazines are a key source of health information. The media are a major source of health information, almost half of women (45%) obtain information about healthy eating from magazines and one in four from TV/radio.[119] Women also obtain information about eating disorders from the media and this may lead to an early awareness that they have a problem. In a recent survey[120] of 120 anorexic women it was found that reading about the characteristics of anorexia nervosa was the most important factor in admitting to having anorexia nervosa, most of the women obtained information from the media, self-help organisations and family or friends.

Annex Three summarises recent work that has been undertaken by the Eating Disorders Association with the media and provides examples of incidents where the media have been used to raise awareness of eating disorders, and have provided useful health information. Since the media have considerable influence in increasing awareness of health issues, it is vital that young women receive the right messages about body shape and healthy weight.

Summary Box

- For eating disorder sufferers, their bodies become the means by which they judge the success of their lives. Encouraging and developing self-esteem which is not dependent upon body size may be a key to protecting vulnerable individuals from developing eating disorders.

- The media can boost self-esteem where it is providing examples of a variety of body shapes, roles and routes of achievement for young men and women. However, it often tends to portray a limited number of body shapes and messages linking external appearance with success — this is potentially damaging to the self-esteem of young people.

- The media is an important source of health care information for young people, particularly through the medium of women's magazines, and their positive contribution to health should not be underestimated. However, it is important that care and consideration is given to the messages that are conveyed by the media and received by young people.

Primary prevention programmes

The goals of primary prevention have been defined as "efforts to eliminate or render ineffective factors involved in the causation of the disorder, and efforts to strengthen the host against noxious influences."[121] In relation to eating disorders it has been stated that "….there is a general need to focus concurrently on reducing pressures for slenderness emanating from media and from family and peers, while somehow enhancing the desire and skills to resist those influences."[89]

How are these goals to be achieved? The pressure on young people could be reduced if more varied examples of body size and shape were presented in the media[122] (hopefully this would also reduce the pressure from peers to conform to an unrealistic body shape) and would require action from media professionals to actively encourage a cultural shift away from an over-emphasis on thinness.[106] Cultural changes in the presentation of the female body and a discouragement of dieting would have a positive impact on all women in Western industrialised societies, and would particularly benefit women vulnerable to eating disorders or chronic dieting.[46] Health promotion campaigns could aim to discourage parents from making weight an issue, and making unhelpful comments about weight to young children and adolescents, which may lead to the young person feeling self-conscious about their body size and shape. Many of these shifts in cultural norms, however, could take a while to 'filter' through and reduce the number of eating disorders.

A more immediate approach may be to take action to 'strengthen the host against noxious influences' (by considering, for example, what cultural aspects apparently provide protection from eating disorders.) Any project aiming to foster the primary prevention of eating disorders would need to consider a number of issues relating to the lives of young people. The following topics for inclusion in educational programmes have been suggested:[123]

- Information about normal physiological, social and psychological changes during puberty, the increased deposition of fat tissue, and the diversity that occurs among individuals;

- Overall nutrition, meal skipping and other eating habits, and the connection between food and emotions;

- Physical activity — its importance and appropriate levels;

- Issues of weight control including an understanding of the physiological and psychological effects of food restriction and chronic dieting, discouragement of drastic weight loss techniques and the facts and myths of dietary fads, realistic and safe methods of weight control, and realistic goals for weight change and maintenance;

- Body image issues, including discussions on the role of the media in suggesting slimness as the answer to social concerns, student images of the ideal body and assistance in determining one's appropriate body weight;

- Women-related issues including the role of women in society, the media's portrayal of women, and the balance between femininity and competence/ autonomy;

- Issues related to autonomy, self-esteem and personal identity;

- Skills for coping with stress and social pressures (ie being assertive);

- Information on anorexia and bulimia nervosa — in a manner in which the 'glamorisation' of these eating disorders is discouraged.

In addition, media literacy programmes have been suggested as a possible way forward for reducing the pressure on young women to be slim; these would include lessons that deconstruct the mass media and assist children in understanding the industry and production of media and help them to question, evaluate and respond thoughtfully to media output such as advertising — Australia recently mandated media education for nearly every student from kindergarten through to grade 12.[124] Careful consideration, however, would need to be given to such programmes in order to ensure that the media is not condemned in a way that simplistically dismissed young people's enjoyment of the media as this may create resistance to engage in critical analyses of media messages.[89]

One example of a recent initiative in the UK is the set of guidelines produced by The City of Liverpool's education and lifelong learning service.[125] The *Guidelines for Schools on Eating Disorders and Body Image* was produced to help schools consider how best to respond to pupils' eating problems and promote a positive self-body image amongst all staff and pupils. It includes a list of resources that can be used to support classroom work and suggestions for incorporating these issues into core curriculum subjects such as English, science, health education and food technology.

Another possible way to strengthen young people's resistance to messages about the importance of appearance could be to find alternative routes of achievement and self-esteem for vulnerable groups who see achieving the proper physical appearance as the only route to acceptance.[126] The Australian study[41] highlights the risk that dieting in adolescent women may give rise to disordered eating. It concludes that women should engage in greater sporting activity. In a recent study, it was found that time to enjoy sports and hobbies is rated by young people as the least important aspect of their lives.[127] There is a concern that certain sporting activities themselves have been associated with an increased risk of developing an eating disorder.[128] This is mainly a problem when the sport is extremely competitive and where a low weight offers performance advantage — for example, gymnastics, swimming and running.[129] Excessive exercising can be a significant component of weight loss in men and women with eating disorders. The prevalence of eating disorders in these individual competitive sports could be explained by the fact that young female athletes often enter competition before they have fully developed secondary sex characteristics. During puberty a previously slender athlete might find that her body is trying to mature, and this may conflict with her training.[129] For the majority of young people who have not developed an eating disorder, however, exercise can be an important component of developing self-esteem and an alternative focus to food, for women wanting to maintain a healthy weight. Another recent study[130] found that women who regularly exercised rated themselves as more attractive, confident, healthy and popular than non-exercisers, although they were significantly heavier than the non-exercising group. There is an increasing body of evidence indicating that "moderate exercise, focusing on mastery rather than aesthetics, can improve perceptions of control, self-esteem and satisfaction with the body",[46] all of which could contribute to a prevention of eating disorders.

In a school situation, low self-esteem can prevent young women from engaging in physical activity, as they may feel self-conscious about their body size or appearance, or they may not be able to afford expensive training shoes or clothing. Young people can be deterred from sporting activity for a variety of reasons including lack of body confidence, lack of nearby facilities, lack of public transport to gymnasiums and sporting facilities, lack of time, cost of activities or sportswear.[131] It has been suggested that "the inability to achieve the aerobics instructor look may leave women feeling defeated, ashamed and desperate".[3] Negative associations with school sport may impact on the future sporting activity, health fitness and self-esteem of young people. The focus of sporting activities and exercise should always be enjoyment, and not the goal of losing weight and achieving a particular body shape. Children who are overweight should not be teased or made self-conscious about their weight in physical education classes and every attempt should be made to include them fully in sporting activities.

As many eating disorders for young women begin at the pubertal developmental stage, more consideration should be given to the particular worries and conflicts that they may experience at this time,[137] and ways of bolstering self-esteem at this vulnerable stage of physical and social development.

It should be noted that much of the research on primary prevention programmes for eating disorders has been conducted in the US, Canada and Australia and evidence of their effectiveness remains uncertain. There is a need for further research to be conducted on the primary prevention of eating disorders in the UK.

Summary Box

- Primary prevention programmes for eating disorders aim to reduce risk factors for the illness and increase young people's resistance to them. Changes can be made at a societal level to achieve these goals, for example, reducing exposure to media images of thin women and increasing awareness of issues relating to body image, self-esteem and pressure to diet, in the school curriculum.

Discussion — the way forward

Anorexia and bulimia nervosa are serious psychiatric illnesses with high mortality and morbidity. Evidence suggests that there are certain genetic predispositions to these illnesses, with environmental factors likely to trigger the illness in vulnerable individuals. In this report we have mainly considered the significant environmental factor of the media, and their role in contributing to low self-esteem and the pressure to diet. We have outlined evidence which suggests that eating disorders became more prevalent in certain periods of history, and in particular cultures, and have examined the possible reasons why eating disorders predominantly affect women, and became prevalent in the late part of the 20th century. We considered that the media play a significant role in the aetiology of eating disorders, although we cannot blame an individual advertisement, television programme or model for their onset, and there is a clear need for more comprehensive research to be conducted on this issue. Children and young adolescents who are in the process of forming their views about their own bodies, and their role in society, are particularly vulnerable to mixed, or confusing messages about healthy eating and desirable body shape.

The effect of the media on social behaviour remains difficult to quantify, and we cannot say with absolute certainty that reducing the number of media images of thin women will necessarily reduce the incidence of disease, at least not in the short term. A wider sociocultural shift may be required to impact greatly on the incidence of disease. This will require the examination of our ideas about beauty and body image in general, and the development of self-esteem in young women. However, if young women are to feel that they are valued for their intrinsic qualities and achievements rather than simply their looks, then we clearly need to address the ways in which contemporary Western culture encourages women to develop a preoccupation with body size and body image, and to perceive weight as their greatest health care concern. We have examined the effect of one component of contemporary culture, the media, as we believe that they are major sources of our cultural ideals. They are not the sole responsible factor for the rise in eating disorders in Western societies since the 1950s-60s. However, they are a factor that we can seek to guide and influence in order to produce better health care outcomes within populations.

Eating disorders are the result of a variety of cultural, environmental and biological influences, but, the precipitant and perpetuating factors of low self-esteem, dieting, and distorted perceptions of healthy body weights are factors which are culturally determined, and are open to change. The media, if they adopt responsible attitudes, can provide valuable health information to young people, and aid the development of high self-esteem and sense of achievement which is not tied to body size. The media, working together with the medical profession, can convey accurate information on healthy body weight and increase awareness of the dangers of dieting in young women. At present, certain sections of the media provide images of extremely thin or underweight women in contexts which suggest that these weights are healthy or desirable. This image contradicts the actual body size of most women in Western industrialised cultures. A more realistic approach to objective body weights — which recognise, for example, that many women are naturally curvaceous or 'pear shaped' and that women's health is endangered by being too thin — is one that should be adopted, for the sake of our young women's health. In addition, it is important to recognise that although this report has focussed mainly on young women — who comprise the majority of sufferers of eating disorders — young men also face the pressure to be physically perfect, and are presented with unrealistic images of how they should look, which may precipitate eating disorders or other unhealthy behaviours such as the abuse of steroids.

It is important that being slightly or moderately overweight is not confused with being obese. Equally, it is a priority that the healthy eating message is not confused with being thin. In a recent survey it was found that almost 60% of clinically underweight women were happy with their weight.[108] Unnecessary worrying over moderate obesity may lead to low self-esteem and depression and associated health risks, particularly if a young woman is teased by her peers. It is particularly important that children who are overweight or obese — or believe that they are — are dealt with in a sensitive manner. In many cases while a child is still developing, a stabilisation of weight may be sufficient to ensure healthy adult weight. This should be achieved by an exercise programme and healthy eating advice. The terms 'diet' and 'dieting' should not be confused — a diet refers to a system of nourishment, dieting is generally regarded as the restriction of food intake.

The goal should not be to demand perfection, or for women to fall into the underweight or lower range of their normal BMI, but for realistic goals to be set, and for upper ranges of 'normal' BMI to be more in evidence on television as role models for young women. It is important that the myth that men find 'stick thin' women attractive is dispelled and that young women realise that there are many acceptable body sizes and shapes, whilst at the same time recognising the health risks of clinically defined obesity. The medical profession itself has been criticised for reinforcing a "hostile cultural attitude which regards even a mild degree of overweight as ugly and abnormal"[52] and it is therefore important that the healthy eating message is not miscommunicated in the form of a thin ideal shape which is unachievable to most naturally curvaceous women.

Recommendations

The Media

1   Broadcasters (or programme makers) and magazine publishers should adopt a more responsible editorial attitude towards the depiction of extremely thin women as role models, and should portray a more realistic range of body images.

2   Producers of TV and printed advertisements should consider more carefully their use of thin women to advertise products, in particular the ITC should review its policy on the use of thin models to advertise products other than slimming aids.

3   Health professionals should work with the television industry to increase awareness of the possible impact of programming on young people, and encourage the inclusion of healthy eating patterns into their programming.

Diet and nutrition

4   Health professionals should work with food manufacturers, and advertising agencies to increase awareness of the key nutritional issues that affect young people. In particular, there should be increased awareness of the impact of faulty nutrition in young adolescents going through puberty.

5   The school curriculum should include the development of critical viewing skills in order to interpret food advertising. Consideration should be given to implementing media literacy programmes, particularly for young children.

6   Health care workers who work directly with children and teenagers must ensure that dieting is not part of a routine unless it is absolutely necessary; it is crucially important that being put on a 'diet' is clearly distinguished from 'dieting' — ie food restriction. Clear, achievable and biologically appropriate targets should be set by heath care professionals if dieting is considered necessary.

Education

7   Schools should have clearly defined anti-bullying policies, and strongly discourage the teasing of overweight children. This should encourage a greater acceptance of normal variation in body size and shape within the population.

8   Schools should develop policies on eating disorders, to enable early detection of the signs and symptoms in children, which could be related to anorexia or bulimia nervosa.

9   School counselling and mentoring services should provide an arena in which young people can address issues of self-esteem, body shape and social popularity.

10 Consideration should be given to the problems faced by young people during physical education classes, eg self-consciousness about body shape, fearing being 'picked last' in a team due to perceived physical unsuitability. Fitness and enjoyment should be considered the key priorities, and children of all body shapes and sizes should be made to feel included in lessons and valued for their contributions, even if they are unable to achieve high levels of success.

Government health strategy

11 The Government's mental health strategy as set out in *Our Healthier Nation* should set clearly defined targets for the reduction in the number of eating disorders, by consideration of preventive measures.

12 There should be increased public education on the connections between dieting, physical activity and health, and health risks associated with eating disorders and being underweight.

13 More resources should be given for mental health services, specifically eating disorder clinics.

Further research

14 The greatest research priority should be given to trials of primary prevention for eating disorders, especially among children and adolescents. These trials should include the provision of a control group, full assessment, optimum follow-up after a reasonable time-lag, with miminum drop-out rates.

15 There should be more research into the subject of the media and possible related effects on children and adolescents, particularly the impact on perceptions of body shape and healthy eating.

16 There should be more research into the 'protective' factors which seem to result in greatly reduced incidence of eating disorders in certain sectors of the population (eg men, certain ethnic minorities).

Annex One:
Symptoms of eating disorders

AN = specific to anorexia nervosa
BN = specific to bulimia nervosa

Food-related features

- Preoccupation with food;

- Spending long periods of time reading cookery books;

- A sensitivity about eating;

- Very restricted eating (AN);

- A preference for eating alone;

- Cooking meals for the family;

- Choosing low-calorie foods to the exclusion of anything else (AN);

- Irritability, distress and arguing, especially around mealtimes and often over small quantities such as whether to eat five or ten peas (AN);

- Strange behaviour around food, such as cutting or crumbling food into pieces, smearing it over the plate, or moving small pieces of food from one part of the plate to another (AN);

- Hiding food under the plate or table, or in serviettes or clothes pockets;

- Leaving the table during the meal, or immediately after, often to go to the bathroom;

- Collecting and storing food;

- Secretive eating;

- Bingeing (BN);

- Vomiting (self-induced);

- Denying hunger when it is obvious that he/she is hungry;

- Measuring self-worth in terms of the amount of food eaten;

- Feeling distressed and guilty about eating;

- Inability to tolerate unplanned events involving food;

- Extreme irritability when meals are earlier or later than usual;

- Using a lot of salt, vinegar or spicy substances (AN);

- Drinking a lot of water (often to make it easier to be sick);

- Drinking a lot of diet cola, or other low-calorie fizzy drinks (to help take away hunger pangs).

General behaviour

There are many other behavioural signs of an eating disorder besides those related specifically to food, eating and mealtimes, which include:

- Frequent weighing;

- Excessive exercising, especially before or after eating, eg walking everywhere, doing a large number of press-ups, repeatedly running up and down stairs, lane swimming, etc;

- Increased willingness to do things involving exercises;

- Gathering information on dieting from leaflets, books and magazines;

- Using laxatives or so-called 'appetite-suppressant' pills;

- Using diuretics ('water pills');

- Wearing baggy clothes (AN);

- Having difficulty sleeping;

- General irritability, especially when questioned about eating;

- Increase in activities unrelated to food, such as homework and sports;

- Increased interest in issues such as starvation in the Third World;

- Increase in attempts to help others, eg doing voluntary work;

- Self-dislike;

- Defiance and stubbornness;

- Development of rigid daily routines;

- Social withdrawal and even isolation;

- Insisting she is fat when it is obvious that she is not overweight;

- Extreme fear of gaining weight;

- Other forms of self-harming, eg scratching, abusing drugs or alcohol.

Physical features

Weight loss, marked fluctuations in weight, purging activities (particularly vomiting and laxative abuse) and excessive exercising all have a number of physical consequences. The most evident of these are:

- Weight loss, which can be quite extreme (AN);

- Weight fluctuations, but generally around average weight (BN);

- Loss of, or failure to start, menstrual periods (BN);

- Dizziness, sometimes fainting;

- Tiredness;

- Stomach pains and feeling full when only small amounts of food have been eaten (AN);

- Low body temperature with a marked tendency to feel the cold (AN);

- Poor temperature control — either too hot or too cold (AN);

- Poor blood circulation leading to cold hands and feet and, if untreated, to sores which don't heal, and can even become ulcerated (AN);

- Skin on hands and feet has a purplish colour;

- Skin generally has a yellowish hue (can arise from eating excessive amounts of carrots);

- Development of fine downy hair on the back (AN);

- Loss of any pubic or underarm hair (AN);

- Head hair becomes dull, lifeless and may fall out;

- Constipation;

- Mouth ulcers and tooth erosion;

- Swollen cheeks (enlargement of the parotid glands, ie those glands that also get swollen in mumps);

- Calluses on the back of the fingers (due to rubbing against the teeth when inducing vomiting);

- Tension headaches.

(Source: Rachel Bryant-Waugh and Bryan Lask. *Eating Disorders: A Parents' Guide*. London:Penguin, 1999)

Annex Two:
Diagnostic criteria for anorexia nervosa and bulimia nervosa

Anorexia nervosa

A	Refusal to maintain body weight at, or above, a minimally normal weight for age and height (eg weight loss leading to maintenance of body weight less than 85% of that expected; or failure to make expected weight gain during period of growth, leading to body weight less than 85% of that expected)
B	Intense fear of gaining weight or becoming fat, even though underweight
C	Disturbance in the way in which one's body weight or shape is experienced; undue influence of body weight or shape on self-evaluation, or denial of the seriousness of the current low body weight
D	In postmenarcheal females, amenorrhoea, ie the absence of at least three consecutive menstrual cycles. (A woman is considered to have amenorrhoea if her periods occur only following hormone, eg, oestrogen, administration)
Specify type:	
Restricting type: during the current episode of anorexia nervosa, the person has not regularly engaged in binge eating or purging behaviour (ie self-induced vomiting or the misuse of laxatives, diuretics, or enemas)	
Binge Eating/Purging type: during the current episode of anorexia nervosa, the person has regularly engaged in binge eating or purging behaviour (ie self-induced vomiting or the misuse of laxatives, diuretics, or enemas)	

Bulimia nervosa

A	Recurrent episodes of binge eating. An episode of binge eating is characterised by both of the following:
	(1) eating, in a discrete period of time (eg within any two hour period), an amount of food that is definitely larger than most people would eat during a similar period of time and under similar circumstances. (2) a sense of lack of control over eating during the episode (eg a feeling that one cannot stop eating or control what or how much one is eating)
B	Recurrent inappropriate compensatory behaviour in order to prevent weight gain, such as self-induced vomiting, misuse of laxatives, diuretics, enemas, or other medications, fasting or excessive exercise
C	The binge eating and inappropriate compensatory behaviours both occur, on average at least twice a week for three months
D	Self-evaluation is unduly influenced by body shape and weight
E	The disturbance does not occur exclusively during episodes of anorexia nervosa
Specify type: **Purging type:** during the current episode of bulimia nervosa, the person has regularly engaged in self-induced vomiting or the misuse of laxatives, diuretics, or enemas	
Nonpurging type: during the current episode of bulimia nervosa, the person has used other inappropriate compensatory behaviours, such as fasting or excessive exercise, but has not regularly engaged in self-induced vomiting or the misuse of laxatives, diuretics, or enemas	

Reprinted with permission from the Diagnostic and Statistical Manual of Mental Disorders, Fourth Edition. Washington DC, American Psychiatric Association, 1994.

Annex Three:
Eating disorders: the media and health information

(This annex has been prepared by the Eating Disorders Association.)

The media can be extremely valuable in raising awareness of eating disorders and in persuading people to seek help and advice.

A notable example was the ITV soap, Emmerdale. In April 1998, the programme scriptwriters contacted the Eating Disorders Association (EDA) requesting information about eating disorders as they were researching a story-line they wished to run about a 14 year old girl with bulimia nervosa.

EDA provided the necessary information and advice and were consulted on the draft scripts. There was concern from both EDA and the producers that the story-line might raise anxiety amongst some viewers and the decision was made to show the EDA helpline numbers after the relevant episodes. EDA agreed to provide additional helpline cover on the evenings when the key episodes were transmitted. (Yorkshire TV kindly assisted with the costs incurred)

The programmes were transmitted during July and August with startling results. On the evening of 29 July, following the end of the programme, 1,771 calls were made to the helpline with another 1,330 calls the following day. On the evening of 8 August, 1,809 calls were received with another 1,528 calls the following day. The next week's episode resulted in 1,048 calls in the evening and 1,153 calls the following day. Over the three week period, nearly 10,000 callers phoned EDA's helplines as a direct result of the programmes.

The latter part of 1999 saw two similar events. EastEnders ran a story about a young girl who in the course of trying to develop a career in modelling, was shown how to vomit in order to control her weight. Following a large number of calls and emails to the BBC, the EDA assisted in constructing a special web site containing information and sources of help for people concerned about the character, or the health of themselves, their family or friends. Again, the BBC ran the helpline number following the next episode and the EDA saw a significant rise in the number of calls to the helpline.

Around the same time, Peak Practice on ITV ran a story-line about over-eating and publicised the helpline number after the programme. Within a few minutes of the episode ending, the helplines were flooded with calls. Even though calls were split between a number of organisations, over the week following the Programme, the EDA received over 9,200 calls for help.

Another recent example of positive media influence was The Tonight programme with Trevor McDonald, broadcast on 20 January 2000. Tracy Shaw, a well known actress in Coronation Street, conducted this part of the programme which was essentially a personal look at the provision of treatment services for eating disorders. The programme highlighted many of the problems people with an eating disorder face in accessing appropriate treatment and help. Again as soon as the helpline number appeared on screen at about 22.30hrs the calls started to flood in, and over the next three days the helpline operators were constantly busy, as over 20,000 people rang EDA.

The news often presents a challenge to EDA, particularly when the death of a high profile celebrity is involved. The death of Diana, Princess of Wales, who had acknowledged a history of bulimia, and was a well-known supporter of EDA, resulted in hundreds of calls from the media and many, many more calls from the public and people affected by an eating disorder. The tragic death of singer, Lena Zavaroni, caused a deluge of media interest and calls for comment from EDA.

Finally, we must remember the influential role that daytime television programmes such as The Tricia Show, Vanessa, and Kilroy play in raising awareness. EDA receives many calls for assistance in finding 'interesting' case studies to be presented and discussed with the audience and other guests on all these shows, calls that the EDA are rarely able to help with, because of concerns for our client group. However many viewers watch these programmes with interest and the producers are kind enough to show our helpline details. As a result many calls from worried or anxious parents and people with an eating disorder are answered, and callers given information and help.

Eating disorders are a real and significant health issue in society today. The surge in media interest and coverage of eating disorders, body image, shape and size over the last two to three years is evidence of the growing concern and interest in these potentially life threatening illnesses. The media can influence both positively and negatively — it is vital that this powerful source of influence is utilised positively.

For help with eating disorders including anorexia and bulimia nervosa contact:

Eating Disorders Association,
First Floor,
Wensum House,
103 Prince of Wales Road,
Norwich, NR1 1DW.

Tel: 01603 621 414 (Helpline — open 9.00am to 6.30pm weekdays)
01603 765 050 (Youthline Callers 18 & under —
open 4.00pm to 6.00pm weekdays)

E-mail: info@edauk.com   *Website:* www.edauk.com

Annex Four: Help information

Information and advice on eating disorders can be obtained from:

- **Anorexia and Bulimia Care**, PO Box 30, Ormskirk, Lancashire, L39 5JR. (A Christian based organisation). *Tel:* 01695 422479. *Website:* www.anorexiabulimiacare.co.uk. *E-mail:* doreen.abc@virgin.net

- **Careline**, The Cardinal Heenan Centre, 326 High Road, Ilford, Essex IG1 1QP. *Tel:* 020 8514 5444 (Office). Counselling Line: 020 8514 1177

- **Centre for Eating Disorders** (Scotland), 3 Sciences Road, Edinburgh, EH9 1LE. *Tel:* 0131 668 3051. *E-mail:* maryamhart@aol.com

- **Eating Disorders Association**, 1st Floor, Wensum House, 103 Prince of Wales Road, Norwich, NR1 1DW. *Tel:* 01603 619090 (Admin), Helpline: 01603 621414. *Website:* www.edauk.com. *E-mail:* info@edauk.com

- **Mental Health Foundation**, 20-21 Cornwall Terrace, London, NW1 4QL. *Tel:* 020 7535 7400. *Website:* www.mhf.org.uk. *E-mail:* mhf@mhf.org.uk

- **Mind**, Granta House, 15-19 Broadway, London E15 4BQ. *Tel*: 020 8519 2122. *Website:* www.mind.org.uk. *E-mail*: contact@mind.org.uk

- **National Centre for Eating Disorders**, 54 New Road, Esher, Surrey, KT10 9NU. *Tel:* 01372 469493. *Fax:* 01372 469550. *Website:* www.eating-disorders.org.uk. *E-mail:* ncfed@globalnet.co.uk

- **Overeaters Anonymous**, PO Box 12863, Bonnyrigg, Edinburgh, EH19 3YF

- **Overeaters Anonymous**, PO Box 19, Stretford, Manchester, M32 9EB. *Tel:* 07000 784985

- **Royal College of Psychiatrists**, 17 Belgrave Square, London, SW1X 8PG. *Tel:* 020 7235 2351. *Website:* www.rcpsych.ac.uk. *E-mail:* rcpsych@rcpsych.ac.uk

- **Sane**, 40 Adler Street, London, E1 1EE. *Tel:* 020 7375 1002 (Admin), *Helpline:* 0345 678000 (12.00 pm — 2.00 pm. 7 days a week. Calls charged at local rate). *Website:* http://osam.mkn.co.uk/help/extra/charity/sane/index

- **The Samaritans**, PO Box 9090, Stirling, SK8 2SA. *Tel:* 0345 909090 (UK), 1850 609090 (Ireland). *Website:* www.samaritans.org.uk. *E-mail:* jo@samaritans.org

- **Turning Point**, New Loom House, 101 Back Church Lane, London E1 4LU. *Tel:* 020 7702 2300. *Website:* www.turning-point.co.uk or www.drugworld.org. *E-mail:* tpmail@turning-point.co.uk

References

1   Harvard Mental Health Letter. www.mentalhealth.com

2   Hsu LKG. *Eating Disorders*. New York: Guildford Press, 1990

3   Striegel-Moore RH, Silberstein LR, Rodin J. Toward an understanding of risk factors for Bulimia. *American Psychologist* 1986;**41**:246-63

4   American Psychiatric Association. *Diagnostic and statistical manual of mental disorders, Fourth Edition*. Washington DC: American Psychiatric Association, 1994

5   British Medical Association. *Understanding Eating Disorders*. London: Family Doctor Publications, 1996

6   Nicholson SD, Ballance E. Anorexia nervosa in later life: an overview. *Hospital Medicine* 1998;**59**:268-72

7   Hall P, Driscoll R. Anorexia in the elderly. *International Journal of Eating Disorders* 1993;**14**:497-9

8   Sharp CW, Freeman CPL. Medical complications of anorexia nervosa. *British Journal of Psychiatry* 1993;**162**:452-62

9   Treasure J, Szmukler G. Medical complications of chronic anorexia nervosa. In: Szmukler G, Dare C, Treasure J, eds. *Handbook of eating disorders: theory, treatment and research*. Chichester: John Wiley and Sons, 1995

10 Keilen M, Treasure T, Schmidt U, Treasure J. Quality of life measurements in eating disorders, angina and transplant candidates: are they comparable? *Journal of the Royal Society of Medicine* 1994;**87**:44-4

11 Brinch M, Isayer T, Tolstrup K. Anorexia nervosa and motherhood: reproductional pattern and mothering behaviour of 50 women. *Acta Psychiatrica Scandinavica* 1988;**77**:98-104

12 Hubert Lacey J, Smith G. Bulimia nervosa: the impact on mother and baby. *British Journal of Psychiatry* 1987;**150**:777-81

13 British Medical Association. *Growing up in Britain: Ensuring a healthy future for our children*. London: BMJ Books, 1999

14 Waugh E, Bulik CM. Offspring of women with eating disorders. *International Journal of Eating Disorders* 1999;**25**:123-33

15 The Mental Health Foundation. *Information Sheet:Eating Disorders*. www.mentalhealth.org.uk/eat.htm

16 Ryan C. Food for Thought. *BMA News Review* 1998;**April 25**:28

17 Myers S, Davies MP, Treasure J. A *General practitioners guide to eating disorders*. Maudsley Practical Handbook Series No2 1993

18 Patton GC. Mortality in eating disorders. *Psychological Medicine* 1988;**18**:947-52

19 Herzog W, Deter HC, Schellberg D, Seilkopf S, Sarembe E, Kroger F, Minne H, Mayer H, Petzold E. Somatic findings at 12 year follow-up of 103 anorexia nervosa patients: results of the Heidelberg-Mannheim follow-up. In: Herzog W, Deter HC, eds. *The course of eating disorders: Long-term follow-up studies of anorexia and bulimia nervosa*. Berlin-Heidelberg: Springer-Verlag, 1992

20 Sullivan PF. Mortality in anorexia nervosa. *American Journal of Psychiatry* 1995;**152**:1073-74

21 Marx RD. Anorexia Nervosa: theories of etiology. In: Alexander-Mott L, Lumsden DB, eds. *Understanding eating disorders: anorexia nervosa, bulimia nervosa and obesity*. Washington: Taylor and Francis, 1994

22   Di Nicola VF. Anorexia Multiforme: self starvation in historical and cultural context: Part I self starvation as a historical chameleon. *Transcultural Psychiatric Research Review* 1990;**27**:165-197

23   Di Nicola VF. Anorexia Multiforme: self starvation in historical and cultural context: Part II anorexia nervosa as a culture-reactive syndrome. *Transcultural Psychiatric Research Review* 1990;**27**:165-197

24   Keesey RE. A set-point theory of obesity. In Brownell KD, Foreyt JP. *Handbook of Eating Disorders: physiology, psychology and treatment of obesity, anorexia and bulimia.* New York: Basic Books,1986

25   Goodwin GM. Neuroendocrine function and the biology of eating disorders. *Human Psychopharmacology* 1990;**5**:249-253

26   Fallon BA, Nields JA. Lyme disease: a neuropsychiatric illness. *American Journal of Psychiatry* 1994;**151**:1571-83

27   Kaye WH, Greeno CG, Moss H, Fernstrom J, Fernstrom M, Lilenfeld LR, Weltzin TE, Mann JJ. Alterations in serotonin activity and psychiatric symptoms after recovery from bulimia nervosa. *Archives of General Psychiatry* 1998;**55**:927-35

28   Holland AJ, Sicotte N, Treasure J. Anorexia nervosa: evidence for a genetic basis. *Journal of Psychosomatic Research* 1988;**32**:561-71

29   Crisp AH. Some possible approaches to prevention of eating and body weight/shape disorders, with particular reference to anorexia nervosa. *International Journal of Eating Disorders* 1988;**7**:1-17

30   Shoebridge P, Gowers SG. Parental high concern and adolescent-onset anorexia nervosa. *British Journal of Psychiatry* 2000;**176**:132-7

31   Raphael FJ, Hubert Lacey J. The aetiology of eating disorders: a hypothesis of the interplay between social, cultural and biological factors. *European Eating Disorders Review* 1994;**2**:143-54

32   Kendler KS, MacLean C, Neale M, Kessler R, Heath A, Eaves L. The genetic epidemiology of bulimia nervosa. *American Journal of Psychiatry* 1991;**148**:1627-37

33   Rende R. Liability to Psychopathology: A Quantitative Genetic Perspective. In: Smolak L, Levine MP, Striegel-Moore R. *The Developmental Psychopathology of Eating Disorders.* New Jersey: Lawrence Erlbaum Associates, 1996

34   Rosen DS, Nuemark-Sztainer D. Review of options for primary prevention of eating disturbances among adolescents. *Journal of Adolescent Health* 1998;**23**:354-63

35   Smolak L, Levine MP. Adolescent Transitions and the Development of Eating Problems. In: Smolak L, Levine MP, Striegel-Moore R. *The Developmental Psychopathology of Eating Disorders.* New Jersey: Lawrence Erlbaum Associates, 1996

36   Russell GFM. The changing nature of anorexia nervosa: an introduction to the conference. *Journal of Psychiatric Research* 1985;**19**:101-9

37   Douglas S. *Where the girls are: growing up female with the mass media.* London: Penguin, 1994

38   Myers A, Rosen JC. Obesity stigmatization and coping: relation to mental health symptoms, body image and self esteem. *International Journal of Obesity* 1999;**23**:221-30

39   Stewart Truswell A. *ABC of Nutrition.* London: BMJ Books, 1999

40   Lattimore PJ, Butterworth M. A test of the structural model of initiation of dieting among adolescent girls. *Journal of Psychosomatic Research* 1999;**46**:295-9

41   Patton GC, Selzer R, Coffey C, Carlin JB, Wolfe R. Onset of adolescent eating disorders, population based cohort study over 3 years. *British Medical Journal* 1999;**318**:765-8

42   Patton GC, Johnson-Sabine E, Wood K, Mann AH, Wakeling A. Abnormal eating attitudes in London schoolgirls - a prospective epidemiological study: outcomes at twelve month follow-up. *Psychological Medicine* 1990;**20**:383-404

43   White JH. Women and eating disorders, Part I: significance and sociocultural risk factors. *Health Care for Women International* 1992;**13**:351-62

44   Hill AJ. Pre-adolescent dieting: implications for eating disorders. *International Review of Psychiatry* 1993;**5**:87-100

45 Kreipe RE, Forbes GB. Osteoporosis: a new morbidity for Dieting Female. *Adolescent Pediatrics* 1990;**86**:478-80

46 Grogan S. *Body Image: understanding body dissatisfaction in men, women and children*. London: Routledge, 1999

47 Crawley H, Shergill-Bonner R. The nutrient and food intakes of 16-17 year old female dieters in the UK. *Journal of Human Nutrition and Dietetics* 1995;**8**:25-34

48 Department of Health. *The Health of Young People 95-97 Volume 1: Findings*. London: HMSO,1998

49 Childress AC, Brewerton TD, Hodges EL, Jarrell MP. The kids eating disorders survey (KEDS): A study of middle school students. *Journal of Academic Adolescent Psychiatry* 1993;**32**:843-50

50 Crawford M, Selwood T. The nutrition knowledge of Melbourne high-school students. *Journal of Food and Nutrition* 1983;**40**:25-34

51 Miller EC, Maropis CG. Nutrition and diet-related problems. *Adolescent Medicine* 1998;**25**:193-210

52 Vandereycken W, Meerman R. Anorexia nervosa: is prevention possible? *International Journal of Psychiatry in Medicine* 1984;**14**:191-205

53 Bemporad JR. Cultural and Historical Aspects of Eating Disorders. *Theoretical Medicine* 1997;**18**:401-20

54 Lasegue EC. De l'anorexie hysterique. *Archives of General Medicine* 1873;**21**:385

55 Gull WW. Anorexia nervosa (apepsia hysterica, anorexia hysterican). *Transactions of the Clinical Society of London* 1874;**7**:22-8

56 Russell GFM. Bulimia nervosa: an ominous variant of anorexia nervosa. *Psychological Medicine* 1979;**9**:429-48

57 Jones D, Fox M, Babigan H, Hutton H. Epidemiology of anorexia nervosa in Monroe County, New York: 1960-1976. *Psychosomatic Medicine* 1980;**42**:551-8

58 Szmulker G, McCance C, McCrone L, Hunter D. Anorexia nervosa: a psychiatric case register study from Aberdeen. *Psychological Medicine* 1986;**16**:49-58

59 Bosch X. Spain tackles eating disorders. *British Medical Journal* 1999;**318**:960

60 Dolan B. Cross-cultural aspects of anorexia nervosa and bulimia: a review. *International Journal of Eating Disorders* 1991;**10**:67-78

61 Ratan D, Ghandi D, Palmer R. Eating disorders in British Asians. *International Journal of Eating Disorders* 1998;**24**:101-5

62 Striegel-Moore R, Smolak L. The role of race in the development of eating disorders. In: Smolak L, Levine MP, Striegel-Moore R. *The Developmental Psychopathology of Eating Disorders*. New Jersey: Lawrence Erlbaum Associates, 1996

63 Powell AD, Kahn AS. Racial Differences in women's desires to be thin. *International Journal of Eating Disorders* 1995;**17**:191-5

64 Furnham A, Alibhai N. Cross cultural differences in the perception of female body shapes. *Psychological Medicine* 1983;**13**:829-37

65 Wang MC, Ho TF, Anderson JN, Sabry ZI. Preference for thinness in Singapore, a newly industrialised country. *Singapore Medical Journal* 1999;**40**:502-7

66 Margo JL. Anorexia nervosa in Males: A Comparison with Female Patients. *British Journal of Psychiatry* 1987;**151**:80-3

67 Hasan MK, Tibbetts RW. Primary anorexia (weight phobia) in males. *Postgraduate Medical Journal* 1977;**53**:146-51

68 Hesse-Biber S. *Am I thin enough yet? The cult of thinness and the commercialisation of identity*. New York: Oxford University Press, 1996

69 Siever M. Sexual orientation and gender as factors in socioculturally acquired vulnerability to body dissatisfaction and eating disorders. *Journal of Consulting and Clinical Psychology* 1994;**62**:252-60

70 Office for National Statistics. *Social Trends 30*. London: The Stationery Office, 2000

71   Neumark-Sztainer D, Story M, Falkner NH, Beuhring T, Resnick MD. Sociodemographic and personal characteristics of adolescents engaged in weight loss and weight/muscle gain behaviors: who is doing what? *Preventive Medicine* 1999;**28**:40-50

72   Paxton SJ, Wertheim EH, Gibbons K, Szmukler GI, Hillier L, Petrovich JL. Body image satisfaction, dieting beliefs and weight loss behaviours in adolescent girls and boys. *Journal of Youth and Adolescence* 1991;**20**:361-79

73   Andersen, Mickalide. Anorexia nervosa in the male: an underdiagnosed disorder. *Psychosomatics* 1983;**24**:1066-75

74   Gordon RA. *Anorexia and Bulimia: Anatomy of a social epidemic.* Oxford: Blackwell, 1990

75   Royal College of Psychiatrists. *Help is at Hand Leaflet 1998 - Anorexia and Bulimia.* www.ex.ac.uk/cimh/help/anorexia.htm.

76   Wolf N. *The Beauty Myth.* Chatto: London, 1990

77   Office for National Statistics. *Social Trends 26.* London: The Stationery Office, 1996

78   Office for National Statistics. *Social Trends 29.* London: The Stationery Office, 1999

79   Lewis MK, Hill AJ. Food advertising on British children's television: a content analysis and experimental study with nine-year olds. *International Journal of Obesity* 1998;**22**:206-14

80   Independent Television Commission. *A spoonful of sugar.* London: Consumers International, 1996

81   Battle EK, Brownell KD. Confronting a rising tide of eating disorders and obesity: treatment vs prevention and policy. *Addictive Behaviors* 1996;**21**:755-65

82   Levine MP, Smolak L. Media as a context for the development of disordered eating. In: Smolak L, Levine MP, Striegel-Moore R. *The Developmental Psychopathology of Eating Disorders.* New Jersey: Lawrence Erlbaum Associates, 1996

83   Dutton B. *The Media.* Harlow: Longman, 1997

84   Lowery SA, De Fleur ML. *Milestones in mass communications research.* New York: Longman, 1995

85   Pearl D, Bouthilet L, Lazar J. *Television and behaviour: ten years of scientific progress and implications for the eighties, 2 vols.* Washington DC: US Government Printing Office, 1982

86   National Food Alliance. *Children: advertisers' dream, nutrition nightmare?* London: National Food Alliance, 1994

87   Dietz WH. You are what you eat - what you eat is what you are. *Journal of Adolescent Health Care* 1990;**11**:76-81

88   Richens ML. Social comparison and the idealised images of advertising. *Journal of Consumer Research* 1991;**18**:71-83

89   Levine MP, Smolak L. The mass media and disordered eating: implications for primary prevention. In: Vandereycken W, Noordenbos G, eds. *The Prevention of Eating Disorders.* Saffron Walden: Athlone Press, 1998

90   Levine MP, Smolak L, Hayden H. The relation of sociocultural factors to eating attitudes and behaviors and behaviors among middle school girls. *Journal of Early Adolescence* 1994;**14**:472-91

91   Silverstein B, Perdue L, Peterson B, Kelly E. The role of the mass media in promoting a thin standard of bodily attractiveness for women. *Sex Roles* 1986;**14**:519-32

92   Andersen AE, DiDomenico L. Diet vs. shape content of popular male and female magazines: a dose-response relationship to the incidence of eating disorders? *International Journal of Eating Disorders* 1992;**11**:283-7

93   Guillen EO, Barr SI. Nutrition, dieting, and fitness messages in a magazine for adolescent women, 1970-1990. *Journal of Adolescent Health* 1994;**15**:464-72

94   Garfinkel DM, Garfinkel PE, Schwartz D, Thompson M. Cultural expectations of thinness in women. *Psychological Reports* 1980;**47**:483-91

95   Brownell KD. Dieting and the search for the perfect body: where physiology and culture collide. *Behaviour Therapy* 1991;**22**:1-12

96   Tiggeman M, Pickering A. Role of television in adolescent women's body dissatisfaction and drive for thinness. *International Journal of Eating Disorders* 1996;**20**:199-203

97   Field AE, Cheung L, Wolf, AM, Herzog DB, Gortmaker SL, Colditz GA. Exposure to the mass media and weight concerns among girls. *Pediatrics* 1999,**103**:E36

98   Pinhas L, Toner BB, Ali A, Garfinkel PE, Stuckless N. The effects of the ideal of female beauty on mood and body satisfaction. *International Journal of Eating Disorders* 1999;**25**:223-6

99   Hamilton K, Waller G. Media Influences on Body Size Estimation in Anorexia and Bulimia: An Experimental Study. *British Journal of Psychiatry* 1993;**162**:837-40

100   Becker AE. *Body, self and society: The View from Fiji.* University of Pennsylvania Press, 1995

101   Craig PL, Swinburn A, Mantega-Smith T, Mantangi H, Vaughan G. Do Polynesians still believe that big is beautiful? Comparison of body size perceptions and preferences of Cook Islands, Maori and Australians. *New Zealand Medical Journal* 1996;**109**:200-3

102   Tolman DL, Debold E. Conflicts of body and image: female adolescents, desire, and the no-body body. In: Fallon P, Katzman MA, Wooley SC. *Feminist Perspectives on Eating Disorders.* New York: Guilford, 1994

103   Bullerwell-Ravar J. How important is body image for normal weight bulimics? Implications for research and treatment. In: Dolan B, Gitzinger I, eds. *Why Women? Gender issues and eating disorders.* London: European Council on Eating Disorders, 1991

104   Attie I, Brooks-Gunn J. Development of eating problems in adolescent girls: a longitudinal study. *Developmental Psychology* 1989;**25**:70-79

105   Myers PN, Biocca FA. The elastic body image: the effect of television advertising and programming on body image distortions in young women. *Journal of Communication* 1992;**42**:108-33

106   Grigg M, Bowman J, Redman S. Disordered eating and unhealthy weight reduction practices among adolescent females. *Preventive Medicine* 1996;**25**:748-56

107   Stice E, Shaw HE. Adverse effects of the media portrayed thin-ideal on women and linkages to bulimic symptomatology. *Journal of Social and Clinical Psychiatry* 1994;**13**:288-308

108   Flour Advisory Bureau Ltd. Bread for Life Campaign. *Pressure to be Perfect.* London,1998

109   Gilbert S, Thompson JK. Feminist explanations of the development of eating disorders: common themes, research findings, and methodological issues. *Clinical Psychology, Science and Practice* 1996;**3**:183-202

110   Sondon-Hagopian N. The Connection between anorexia nervosa and achievement in modern society - a review Progress. *Family Systems Research and Therapy* 1992;**1**:71-82

111   Button EJ, Sonuga-Barke EJS, Davies J, Thompson M. A prospective study of self-esteem in the prediction of eating problems in adolescent schoolgirls: Questionnaire findings. *British Journal of Clinical Psychology* 1996;**35**:193-203

112   American Society of Plastic and Reconstructive Surgeons. *Average surgeon fees, 1996.* Arlington Heights IL: American Society of Plastic and Reconstructive Surgeons, 1997

113   Morgan JF, Lacey JH. Smoking, eating disorders and weight control (Letter). In: *Postgraduate Medical Journal* 1999;**75**:127

114   Marcus BH, Albrecht AE, King TK, Parisi AF, Pinto BM, Roberts M, Niaura RS, Abrams DB. The efficacy of exercise as an aid for smoking cessation in women: a randomized controlled trial. *Archives of Internal Medicine* 1999;**159**:1229-34

115   Hill AJ. Impossible Expectations. In: *Signpost* (the Eating Disorders Association Newsletter) December 1996;p2

116   Wilkinson H. *Addicted to perfection. Young people's notions of success.* Speech to launch the Bread for Life Campaign, 13 July 1999

117   Basow SA, Kobrynowicz D. What is she eating? The effects of meal size on impressions of a female eater. *Sex Roles* 1993;**28**:335-44

118   Finch H, White C. *Physical activity: what we think. Qualitative research among women aged 16 to 24.* London: Health Education Authority, 1998

119   Flour Advisory Bureau Ltd. Bread for Life Campaign. *Research summary.* London, 1999

120   Noordenbos G. Important factors in the process of recovery according to patients with anorexia nervosa. In: Herzog W, Deter HC, eds. *The Course of Eating Disorders: Long-term follow-up studies of anorexia and bulimia nervosa.* Berlin: Springer-Verlag, 1992

121   Striegel-Moore RH, Steiner-Adair C. Primary prevention of eating disorders: further considerations from a feminist perspective. In: Vandereycken W, Noordenbos G, eds. *The Prevention of Eating Disorders.* Saffron Walden: Athlone Press, 1998

122   Slade P. Prospects for prevention. In: Szmukler G, Dare C, Treasure J. *Handbook of eating disorders: theory, treatment and research.* Chichester: John Wiley and Sons, 1995

123   Neumark-Sztainer D. Excessive weight preoccupation: Normative but not harmless. *Nutrition Today* 1995;**30**:68-74

124   Strasburger VC, Donnerstein E. Children, adolescents and the media: issues and solutions. *Pediatrics* 1999;**103**:129-39

125   City of Liverpool Education and Lifelong Learning Service. *Guidelines for schools on eating disorders and body images.* Liverpool Health Promotion Service: Liverpool, 2000

126   Ewell F, Smith S, Karmel MP, Hart D. The sense of self and its development: a framework for understanding eating disorders. In: Smolak L, Levine MP, Striegel-Moore R. *The Developmental Psychopathology of Eating Disorders.* New Jersey: Lawrence Erlbaum Associates, 1996

127   Flour Advisory Bureau Ltd. Bread for Life Campaign. Press Release. *Young women are adopting a male model of success new Bread for Life research shows.* London, 1999

128   Lindeman AK. Quest for ideal weight: costs and consequences. *Official Journal of the American College of Sports Medicine* 1999;**31**:1135-40

129   Palmer RE, Frost CM. Eating disorders in female athletes: A literature review for the chiropractic sports physician. *Chiropractic Sports Medicine* 1994;**8**:10-17

130   Furnham A, Titman P, Sleeman E. Gender and locus of control correlates of body image dissatisfaction. *European Journal of Social Behaviour and Personality* 1994;**8**:183-200

131   Health Education Authority. *Physical activity - what we think - qualitative research among women aged 16-24.* London: HEA, 1998

132   Friedman SS. Girls in the 90s: A gender-based model for eating disorder prevention. *Patient Education and Counselling* 1998;**33**:217-24